JOURNEYS FROM WITHIN

52 Short Visualizations

Mark Deith

Dedicated to Sheila, my loving wife and muse.

ABOUT THIS BOOK

Welcome to a collection of 52 visual journeys, each crafted to guide you toward a sense of peace, relaxation, and harmony. These stories are designed to grow with you—beginning with shorter reflections that take just a minute or two, gradually unfolding into deeper, more immersive tales that span up to ten minutes.

Each journey takes place in a unique environment, often inspired by the beauty of the natural world. From serene forests to sunlit meadows, from tranquil waters to starlit skies, these settings are meant to transport you to places that soothe your soul and spark your imagination.

Some of these visualizations carry uplifting messages or gentle moral insights, inviting you to reflect on themes like self-acceptance, gratitude, or love. Others exist simply to provide an escape in a moment of quiet.

The intention behind this collection is simple yet profound: to bring moments of calm into your life, to ease the mind, and to nurture a deeper connection with yourself and the world around you. Whether you're seeking a brief respite from a busy day or a deeper exploration of inner peace, these stories are here to accompany you on your journey.

So find a comfortable space, take a deep breath, and let your mind wander. With each page, allow yourself to let go, unwind, and be fully present in the moment. The journey is yours to take—step by step, word by word.

HOW TO USE THIS BOOK

This book is a collection of guided journeys designed to bring relaxation, spark creativity, and offer moments of introspection. Whether you're an individual seeking a peaceful escape, a yoga teacher guiding students through meditation or savasana, or someone leading a group in a moment of calm, these visualizations are crafted to adapt to your needs.

For Individuals:
Enjoy these visualizations during quiet moments, perhaps as part of your morning routine, before bed, or whenever you need to reset and reconnect. Each story invites you to immerse yourself in its vivid scenes, allowing your mind to unwind and your spirit to recharge.

For Yoga Teachers:
The stories have a yoga-inspired flair and are perfect for use in meditation & savasana, or as part of a themed class. They can help your students transition into stillness, deepen their practice, or simply leave with a sense of calm and inspiration.

For Group Settings:
These journeys can be a powerful tool in classrooms, workshops, or community groups to foster mindfulness and unity. They are versatile and accessible, providing a shared journey that encourages both personal reflection and collective peace.

Each visualization is intentionally neutral—free of political, religious, or inappropriate messaging. They aim to be universally welcoming, allowing anyone, regardless of background or belief, to find relaxation and connection. To ensure a broader audience can enjoy this book, it is written in American English.

How to Begin:
Feel free to explore the stories in any order. Start with a shorter visualization for a quick moment of calm, or dive into a longer journey when you have time to truly immerse yourself. Read them aloud or in silence, and adjust the pacing to suit your needs.

The ultimate intention of this book is simple: to provide a sanctuary for your mind and heart. May these journeys bring you peace, inspire your imagination, and remind you of the beauty both within and around you.

NEW TO MEDITATION?

Meditation is a simple yet powerful practice that invites you to be fully present in the moment. In our busy, often chaotic lives, it's easy to get caught up in thoughts about the past or worries about the future. Mindfulness gently guides you back to the here and now, helping you cultivate a sense of calm, clarity, and acceptance.

At its core, mindfulness is about paying attention—deliberately and without judgment—to your thoughts, feelings, bodily sensations, and the surrounding environment. It's not about silencing the mind or achieving a state of perfect peace. Instead, it's about noticing whatever arises with curiosity and compassion, letting go of any need to control or change it.

To begin a mindfulness practice, find a quiet space where you can sit comfortably. Close your eyes or soften your gaze and take a few slow, deep breaths. Focus your attention on the sensation of your breath as it moves in and out of your body. Feel the rise and fall of your chest, the coolness of the air as you inhale, and the warmth as you exhale.

Inevitably, your mind will wander. This is completely normal. When you notice your attention has drifted, gently bring it back to your breath or the point of focus you've chosen. This act of returning—again and again—is the essence of mindfulness.

With regular practice, mindfulness meditation can bring a sense of balance and resilience to your daily life. It encourages self-awareness, reduces stress, and can even enhance creativity and problem-solving.

In the pages that follow, you'll encounter guided visualizations that integrate elements of mindfulness. These journeys are designed to help you relax, explore your inner world, and find peace in the present moment. Whether you're new to mindfulness or looking to deepen your practice, let these stories be a gentle guide on your path to well-being.

May these pages bring you moments of calm, inspiration, and connection. Enjoy the journey, and may peace and light guide you every step of the way.

I
Day at the Races

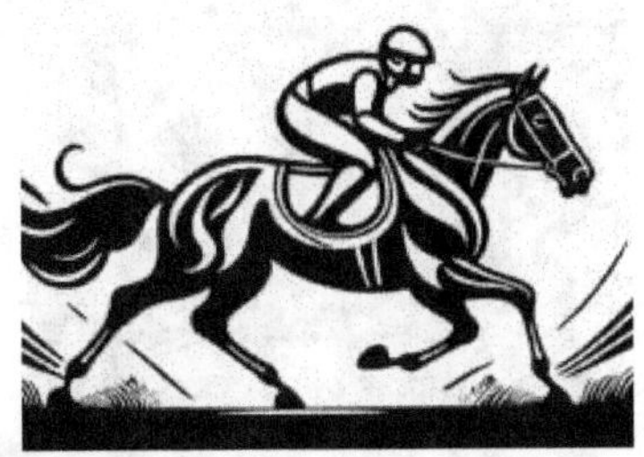

Imagine yourself standing on a grand balcony overlooking a bustling racecourse on raceday. Around you, there's a crowd of elegantly dressed people - refined, polished, maintaining their appearances. The conversations are quiet, and the air is filled with sophistication, but there's also a sense of distance. As you look closer you notice everyone is wearing masks, deliberately hiding who they really are.

Now, shift your gaze down below to where there's another group of people, much more relaxed, laughing freely, unconcerned with how they look and without masks. Their movements are unrestrained, their joy effortless, and there's no need to perform or fit into any mold.

Take a moment to feel the contrast between these two groups. Where do you feel most at ease? Do you feel pulled toward the formality of the balcony or the carefree energy below? Or maybe you find your place somewhere in between.

With each inhale, imagine stepping toward the space where you feel most at home, where you can authentically be yourself. And with each exhale, let go of the need to conform to anyone else's standards.

II

Shelves of Wisdom

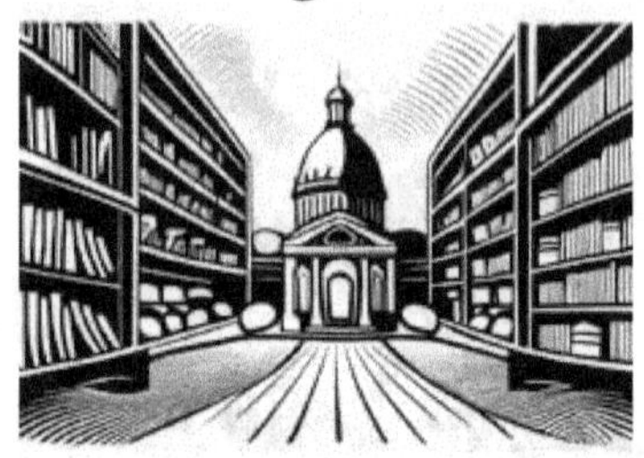

Close your eyes and take a few deep breaths, allowing yourself to settle into the stillness. Imagine stepping into a beautiful, ancient library, a place that feels timeless and wise. The shelves are lined with books of knowledge, each one filled with insights from those who've walked the path before you. The air is calm, the space serene, and soft light filters through high, arched windows.

As you walk quietly through the rows of books, the gentle sound of your footsteps is the only noise. You feel a deep sense of peace, as if this library has always been here, waiting for you.

You find a comfortable chair in a quiet corner, and you sit down. Before you is an open book, but as you look closer, you realize this book is your own. Its pages are blank, waiting to be filled with the wisdom that already lives inside you.

In the stillness, you connect with your inner teacher - the quiet voice within that holds all the answers you seek. You take a deep breath, knowing this place of wisdom is always within you, waiting for you to return.

III

Starry Night

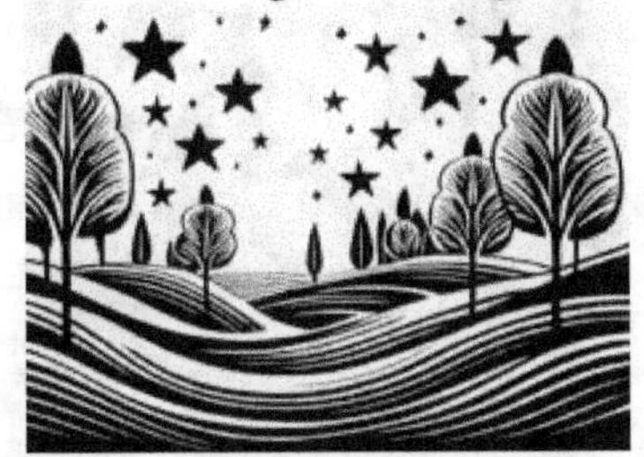

Now, gently bring yourself to a peaceful place and visualize yourself outside at night. You're lying on your back on the cool earth beneath you, the air still. It's dark, very dark, so dark that you can barely see your hand in front of you. But as you settle, you begin to notice tiny pinpricks of light piercing through the darkness. Stars. More and more begin to appear, until above you stretches the vast, glittering expanse of the Milky Way.

You feel calm, connected to the stillness, and then something magical happens. The sky begins to change, a wave of green light flickers on the horizon. The aurora borealis. It dances across the sky in shimmering greens, reds, and purples, each wave more beautiful than the last. The light swirls and moves, filling the night with energy, reminding you that even in the darkest moments, light is always there, sometimes hidden, but always present.

Feel this light - this power - within you. With every breath, imagine the waves of the aurora filling you with peace and balance. The light has overcome the darkness, and you are part of that harmony.

The Weight of Reflection

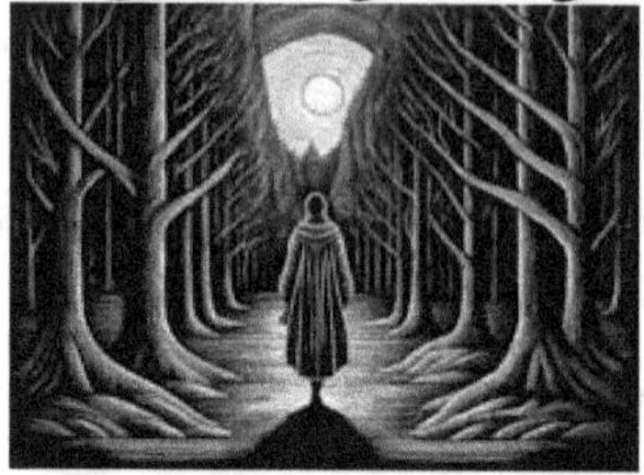

Picture being at home feeling tense and seeking calm, peace, and balance, you opt for meditation. Alone, with a hopeful twenty-minute window of solitude, you settle on the sofa, legs crossed, back straight, hands in the dhyana mudra (rest your hands on your lap, palms facing upwards. Place your right hand on top of your left hand, with your fingers extended). Closing your eyes, you inhale slowly through the nose, exhaling from the mouth. As usual, you tune into surrounding sounds, the ticktock of a clock on the mantelpiece, occasional passing cars (and no annoying family). Concentrating on your breath, you feel relaxation wash over you.

However, your mind wanders briefly to a memory from years ago, a source of shame. It was a moment you're not particularly proud of, a chapter in your life that occasionally resurfaces, bringing with it feelings of regret and discomfort. Despite the passing years and personal growth, the weight of that memory lingers, casting a shadow over your present peace.

Life is made up of fleeting moments, each one precious and unique. Regrets about the past and worries about the future can cloud our vision and steal the joy of the present. The past can't be changed, and the future is still unwritten. By embracing the present, we free ourselves from the weight of yesterday and the uncertainties of tomorrow. In the now, we find clarity and the freedom to truly live. So, let's focus on today, cherish each moment, and experience life to its fullest.

V
Whispering Canopy

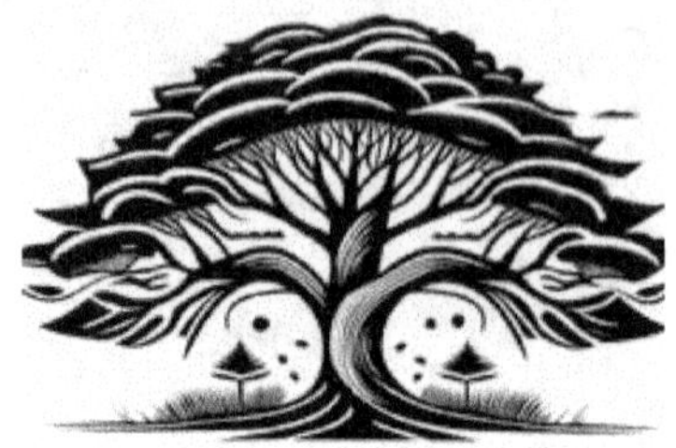

Feel the earth beneath you, solid and supportive, as you sit grounded and present. In your mind's eye, imagine yourself walking into a peaceful forest. The air is crisp and fresh, filled with the scent of pine and floral aromas. Tall trees tower above you, their branches swaying gently with the breeze, offering shade and protection.

You come upon a magnificent tree, its trunk wide and strong, its roots stretching deep into the earth. This tree invites you to sit beneath it, to connect with its ancient wisdom. As you settle into your seat, feel the tree's energy, steady and grounding. Imagine its roots reaching through the earth, anchoring you, while its branches extend high toward the sky, open and free.

As you breathe, draw in the energy of the tree, letting it fill you with a sense of stability, calm, and strength. With each exhale, release any tension, letting it drift away on the breeze. You are supported, connected to both the earth and the sky, just like the tree.

Now, imagine yourself gently flowing through your yoga practice beneath this tree, each movement guided by nature's rhythm. Feel a sense of ease and gratitude for your body, rooted and free, just like this tree.

When you're ready, slowly begin to bring your awareness back to this moment, carrying the peace and balance of the forest within you.

VI

Golden Light

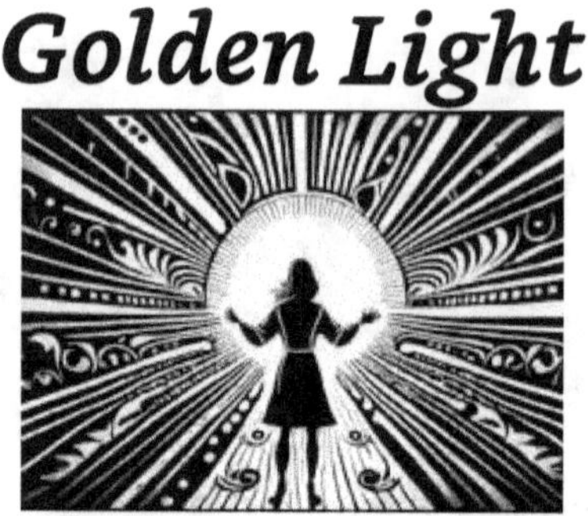

As you settle into this moment, release the urge to evaluate or critique. Let go of any expectations about what your practice "should" look like and instead turn your attention inward. Focus on the feeling of simply being here, now, in this body—just as it is, without judgment or comparison.

Picture a warm, golden light glowing softly at the center of your chest, steady and reassuring. This light symbolizes pure love and unconditional acceptance. As you inhale deeply, feel this light expand, growing brighter and radiating outward through every part of your being. With each breath, it softens any tension, soothes areas of discomfort, and fills you with a profound sense of peace and wholeness.

As this light expands, imagine it wrapping you in a comforting embrace, a reminder that you are enough just as you are. Allow it to guide you through your practice, reminding you that your body, in all its strength and uniqueness, is worthy of love and gratitude.

Feel appreciation for the way your body supports you in every moment, for the breath that sustains your life, and for the personal journey that has brought you to this very moment. This is your time, your space, and your sanctuary.

With each inhale, draw in acceptance, letting it fill your heart. With each exhale, release love—love for yourself, love for this moment, love for the present experience. Let this breath-centered awareness carry you forward as we begin our warm-up, cultivating gratitude and light within you.

VII

A Day of Light

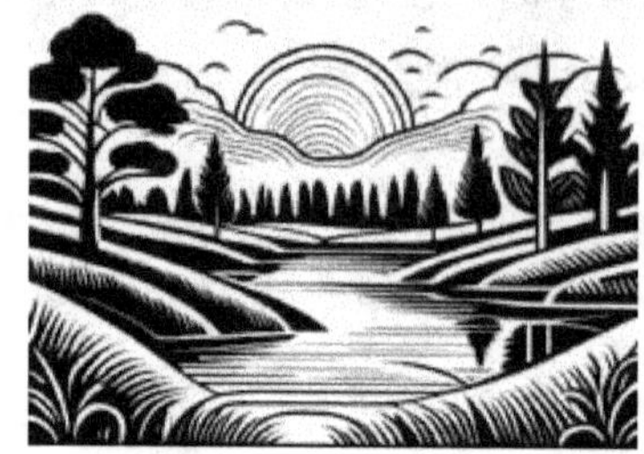

Exhale deeply and feel yourself grounding into the earth, fully connected to the energy of the season. Picture yourself standing in a wide, sun-drenched field beneath a vast, brilliant blue sky that seems to stretch forever. The sun, warm but not overbearing, caresses your skin, wrapping you in its golden glow like a gentle embrace. Around you, the colors of summer are softening; the once-vivid greens of the grass and trees fading into richer, more muted tones. Wildflowers sway lazily in the breeze, their delicate petals releasing one by one, carried off like tiny messengers of the changing season.

Close your eyes for a moment and immerse yourself in the sounds of this tranquil scene. Hear the faint rustling of leaves as the wind weaves through the trees, the soft hum of insects lingering in the air, and the occasional call of a distant bird. These are the sounds of summer gently winding down, a symphony of nature preparing for rest.

Feel the stillness that accompanies the end of the season; a profound, quiet celebration of the growth, vibrancy, and life that summer has nurtured. Let this stillness settle into your own heart, offering a moment of reflection and gratitude.

As the sun begins its descent, painting the sky with streaks of amber and crimson, it casts long, golden shadows across the field.

Breathe in deeply and gather the gifts of summer—its energy, its light, and its abundance. Feel these gifts filling you with warmth and strength, preparing you to carry them forward into the cooler, quieter months ahead.

VIII

Among the Silent Giants

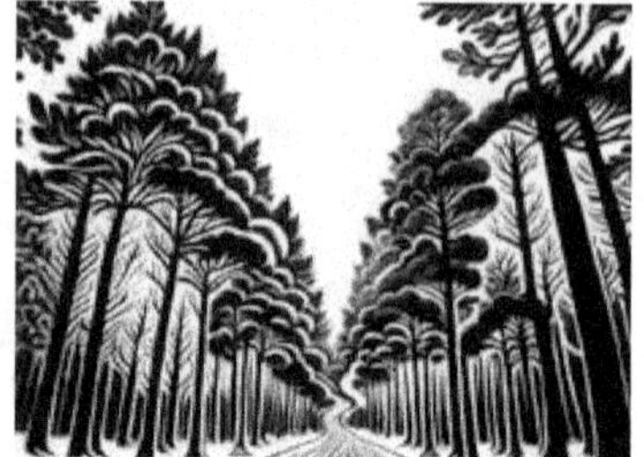

Imagine yourself standing at the edge of a serene forest. The scent of pine and earth fills the air, and dappled sunlight filters through the canopy, casting a gentle glow around you. As you take a step forward, a sense of tranquility envelops you.

Picture yourself following a well-trodden path into the heart of the forest. With each step, you feel more connected to the natural world around you. The sound of birds singing and leaves rustling in the breeze creates a soothing symphony that calms your mind.

As you walk, you come across a small clearing. In the centre stands a majestic tree, its branches reaching towards the sky. You feel drawn to it, sensing the wisdom and strength it embodies. Find a comfortable spot beneath its branches, and sit down, feeling the solid ground beneath you.

Visualize yourself unrolling a yoga mat and sitting down, feeling grounded and connected to the earth beneath you. You are surrounded by nature's beauty, each element contributing to a sense of harmony and balance. Acknowledge any doubts or fears you might have, seeing them as small pebbles. With each deep breath, imagine gently placing these pebbles on the ground, where they dissolve into the earth, leaving you feeling lighter and more at ease.

Now, see yourself moving gracefully through your yoga practice. Each pose flows effortlessly into the next, your body and mind working in perfect harmony. You feel strong, capable, and empowered. The forest around you enhances your sense of calm and focus, and you feel a deep connection to the natural world.

You belong here, in this serene space, and this is your time to grow and flourish.

IX

The Tranquil Garden

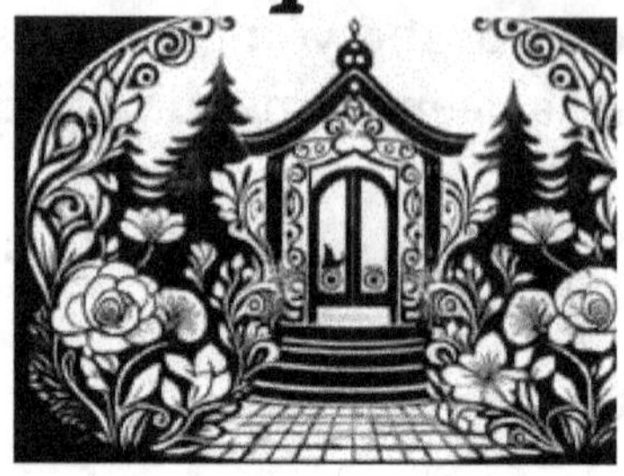

Close your eyes and take a deep breath. Imagine you're walking into a yoga class at a hall. The air is filled with the calming aromas from a scent diffuser and soft Indian music plays in the background. You unroll your mat and settle into a comfortable position.

As the class begins, the instructor guides you into a visualization. Picture yourself in a beautiful, tranquil garden, surrounded by lush greenery and vibrant flowers. The sun is shining warmly, and you feel a gentle breeze on your skin.

As you breathe deeply, imagine the air filling your lungs with positivity and peace. With each exhale, release any tension or stress.

In this garden, you find a comfortable spot to sit and meditate. Feel the earth beneath you, solid and supportive. As you focus on your breath, imagine roots growing from your body into the ground, grounding you and connecting you to the earth's energy.

Now, visualize a soft, warm light beginning to glow within you, starting at your center and expanding outward. This light represents your inner strength and calm. Let it grow, filling your entire being with warmth and empowerment.

Take another deep breath, and as you exhale, let go of any lingering doubts or fears. Feel yourself becoming lighter, more relaxed, and completely at peace.

Gradually, bring your awareness back to the hall. Feel the mat beneath you and the energy of the room around you. Know that you can carry this sense of calm and strength with you, both on and off the mat.

When you're ready, slowly open your eyes, feeling refreshed and empowered, ready to embrace the rest of the class with a positive and peaceful mindset.

Drift and Dream

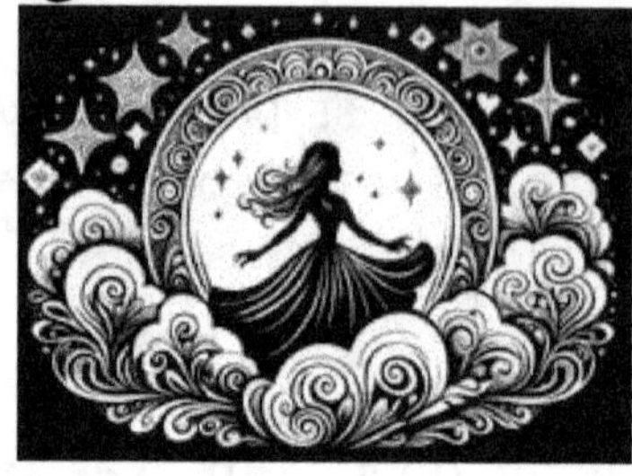

I would like you to imagine that you are floating on a soft, fluffy white cloud. Feel the surface beneath you becoming softer and more cloud-like, which is rising out of the floor you are on, surrounding you in it's protective support as you float on upwards.

Feel the cloud beneath you, reassuringly secure. It's almost like floating in the air as you sink into it. It is a wonderful feeling. Your cloud can float wherever you choose. It is very safe and very calming.

It's a beautiful day as you continue floating, drifting, rising even higher if you wish. The ground below you looks like a patchwork quilt. Green grass. Golden fields and blue patches of rivers and lakes. You can even see the shadow of your own cloud.

You can float wherever you like and look down on forests, beaches, over seas or perhaps you would like to drift in between the rocky peaks of mountains. Wherever you choose, enjoy that place. If you grow tired, lie back, sink into the cloud and feel the warmth of the golden light from the sun.

Now it is time to return to your day. Let your cloud take you there. Feel it flying through the sky, back to where you need to go, and let it lower you down, back toward the ground, back to where you were. Let the cloud blend with the floor and feel it slowly disappear as the real surface becomes more solid beneath you.

Gradually come back to the present. Feel the mat below you. Become more and more aware and alert. Open your eyes when you are ready and look around. See your surroundings as our body awakens after your journey floating on a cloud.

XI

By the Edge

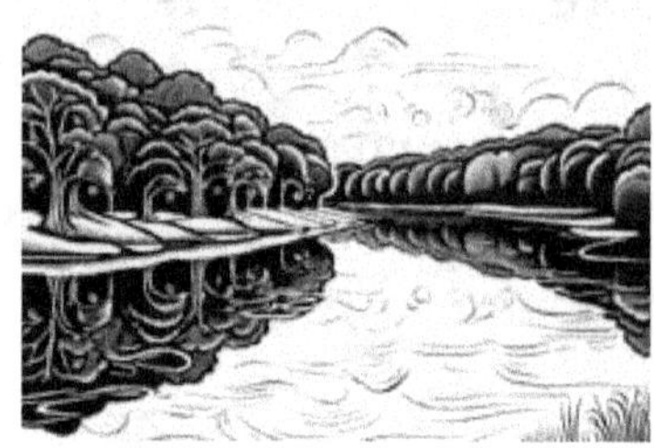

Allow yourself to drift into a scene where you are standing at the edge of a serene riverbank. The air is cool and fresh, filled with the subtle scent of damp earth and distant wildflowers. You can hear the gentle, rhythmic sound of water as a wide river flows smoothly in front of you, its surface shimmering softly in the sunlight. The river moves with a calm, continuous current, carrying leaves, twigs, and delicate branches downstream in a graceful, effortless dance.

In your hand, imagine you're holding a small object, something symbolic of a thought, a worry, or an attachment that has lingered with you. This could be something familiar, perhaps a smooth stone or a light feather—whatever feels right to represent this connection. Take a moment to feel its weight in your palm, the contours and textures beneath your fingertips. Notice any attachment you have to this object, whether it's a strong, tangible pull or a subtle reluctance.

After a quiet moment, take a deep breath, and with gentle intention, extend your hand over the water. Slowly, you release the object into the river. Watch as it rests briefly on the surface before being swept away by the current, moving further and further downstream, fading from view with each gentle ripple.

As it drifts away, allow yourself to feel a sense of release, a lightness that comes from letting go of what no longer serves you. You trust the flow of the river to carry it exactly where it needs to go, beyond your sight and beyond your concern.

Now, as you breathe in, invite in a fresh sense of spaciousness and renewal. With each inhale, let in new energy, clarity, and ease. You are lighter, unburdened, and open to the calm flow of the present moment.

XII

Ujjayi

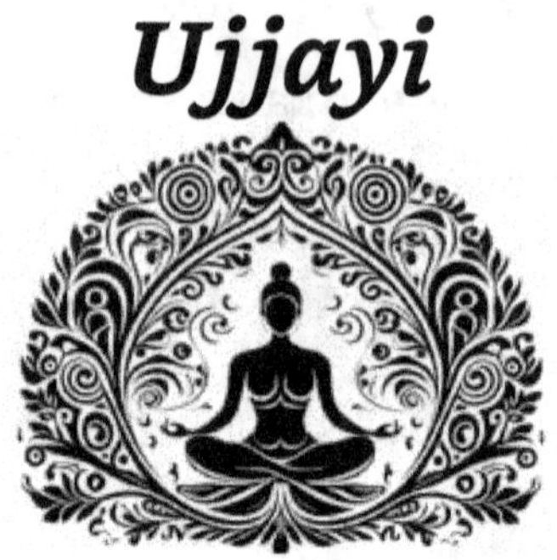

Feel the world around you fade as you step gently and shift your attention inward. Begin to breathe deeply in and out through your nose, and as you do, start to lightly constrict the back of your throat. With this slight narrowing, your breath takes on a soft, whispering sound, like the murmur of waves rolling against a distant shore. This is the breath of Ujjayi, the "Victorious Breath," known for its calming, steadying effect—a breath that draws you into presence.

With each inhale, imagine yourself standing on the edge of an endless, tranquil beach. The sky above is painted in soft shades of morning, a gentle warmth from the sun brushes your skin, and the sand beneath your feet is cool and powder-soft, grounding you to the earth. As you breathe in, the waves advance toward the shore, their quiet power carrying a sense of calm and clarity that fills your entire being. With each exhale, the waves retreat, drawing back into the vastness, carrying away any tension, any remnants of worry or restlessness. Feel a lightness in your chest as you let each wave dissolve what you no longer need.

You are here, in perfect rhythm with the ocean's dance, your breath rising and falling like the tide. There is something timeless in this cycle, as if you are not simply on a beach, but part of an ancient flow that has existed since the beginning of time. Just as waves have carved the shore for eons, this breath carves space within you—space to release, space to receive, and space to simply be.

Let this steady, oceanic breathing become an anchor, a guide, holding you in a state of ease and strength. Feel how the sound of your breath echoes the sound of the sea, a reminder of nature's power and its gentle rhythm.

The ocean breath is a reminder of the resilience that exists within you, a reminder that calmness, like the shore, is ever-present, always there to return to. As you inhale, draw in peace and calm; as you exhale, release anything that weighs heavy, trusting that the waves will carry it away.

XIII

Nature's Palette

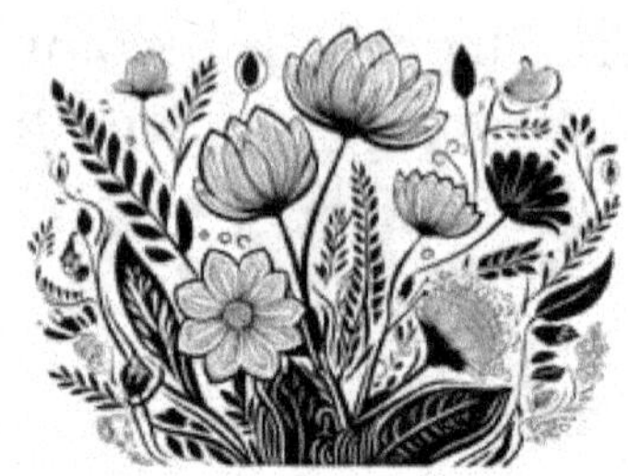

Take a deep breath, and imagine yourself standing at the edge of a vast, open meadow. The air is fresh, carrying a gentle, earthy fragrance mixed with the scent of wildflowers. Step forward into this meadow, and feel the soft grass beneath your feet, grounding you, connecting you to the earth.

As you settle here, take in the vibrant scene before you. Each flower in this meadow is unique, a dazzling array of colors, shapes, and textures. There are tall, regal sunflowers reaching toward the sky, delicate daisies swaying in the breeze, and bright red poppies nestled close to the earth. Some flowers are bold and bright, others are soft and subtle, yet all are equally beautiful in their own way. Each flower is thriving in its space, blooming without hesitation, embracing its own shape, color, and form.

Find a spot to rest, perhaps lying down among the flowers or sitting in the grass. Feel the warmth of the sun above, bathing everything in a golden light that brings out the vivid colors around you. Notice the way the flowers move gently with the breeze, unbothered by the world around them, simply existing as they are meant to.

Take a moment to breathe deeply, and let the peaceful energy of this meadow fill you. Just as each flower here is different yet belongs, you too belong exactly as you are. Like these flowers, you have your own unique strengths, colors, and qualities that contribute to the beauty of the world. There is no need to change or hide; you are enough, just as you are.

As you close your eyes and inhale, feel yourself absorbing the meadow's energy, letting it remind you of your own individuality. And with each exhale, let go of any pressure to conform or compare. In this moment, like the flowers, you are free to embrace your own beauty and uniqueness, to stand tall or simply rest in your own way.

When you're ready, take a last look at this vibrant field, knowing you can return to it anytime you need a reminder that you, too, are a unique and beautiful part of this world.

XIV

Message in a Bottle

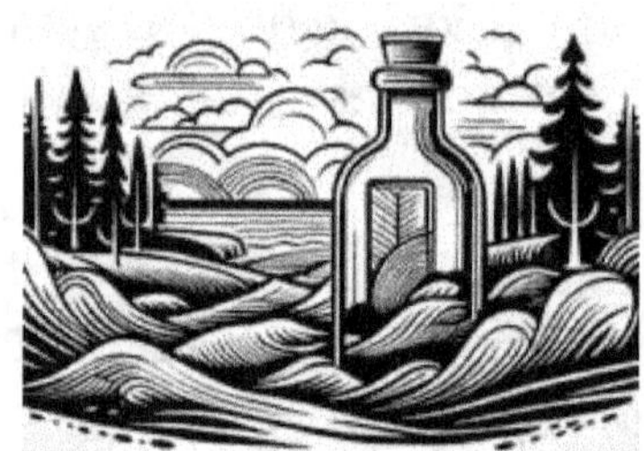

Take a moment to settle into your breath, letting it become steady and easy. Now, imagine yourself standing on a peaceful bridge that stretches over a gently flowing river. The water below you is calm yet determined, moving steadily downstream. You lean on the bridge railing, gazing down into the river's depths, and think about the journey that anything placed into this flow might take.

Picture yourself holding a small glass bottle with a message rolled up inside. You think of tossing it into the river and letting it be carried along by the water. You watch in your mind as the bottle begins its journey downstream, floating smoothly along. Imagine how, bit by bit, the river widens, eventually merging with other waterways, becoming stronger, and gathering force as it heads toward the open sea.

Now, envision the bottle reaching the ocean, a vast expanse where waters mingle and currents shift. You realize that it might travel thousands of miles, perhaps reaching distant shores you may never see. Maybe one day, a stranger will come across this bottle, discovering your message or perhaps the picture you decided to include instead, something universal that might be understood by anyone. In this way, you feel a connection with people far beyond your sight.

As you stand on the bridge, you feel a sense of kinship with this unknown person, who might one day pick up the bottle and understand something about you through its contents. You recognize that we all share the same currents of life, and that the boundaries of distance or culture are softened by our shared experiences.

This thought brings you back to moments in meditation when you feel connected, as though people all over the world, even those far away, might be sharing the same practice, breathing and being present. Allow this feeling of connection to settle within you, bringing a sense of belonging, knowing that we are never as isolated as we might think.

Breathe in this awareness of connectedness, and as you exhale, feel any sense of separateness dissolve, leaving only peace. Take a few more breaths here, knowing that this river, like life itself, connects us all.

XV

Reflection

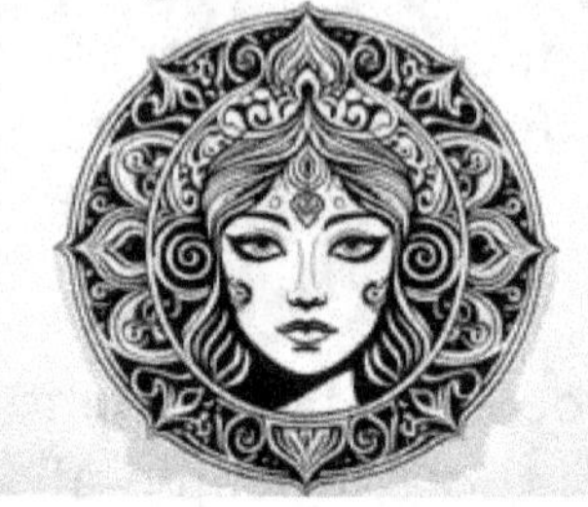

Imagine yourself standing before a tall, beautifully framed mirror, set in a quiet, serene space. The room is softly lit, with gentle, warm light casting a glow around you. This mirror is no ordinary reflection; it holds a depth that feels almost alive, capturing not just your outer form but the entirety of who you are - your thoughts, your emotions, your experiences, the layers of life you've accumulated over the years.

Take a slow, deep breath and let your eyes meet your own reflection. Take this moment to simply observe without any judgment or critique. Look beyond the surface. You see someone standing before you who has overcome challenges, embraced moments of joy, and continued to grow, no matter what life has brought. This person looking back at you is complex, resilient, and full of stories.

As you breathe in deeply, let a soft, warm feeling of acceptance wash over you, flowing from head to toe. Accept yourself entirely as you are in this very moment, with no need to change anything at all. Every part of you, every thought, every experience, has brought you to thismoment, and that's more than enough. Feel the peacefulness of this acceptance filling you.

With each gentle breath out, feel any lingering self-criticism, doubts, or worries dissolve and fade, as though they're melting into the air around you. Let them drift away, replaced by a growing sense of ease and inner calm.

Now, visualize yourself stepping closer to the mirror, feeling a sense of connection deepen as you do. Slowly, you raise a hand and place it gently on the cool surface of the mirror. Through this touch, you're connecting with the image in front of you - a person worthy of kindness, compassion, and understanding. You are deserving of love, just as you are. Let this truth settle warmly within you.

Take one last deep breath, breathing in that feeling of worthiness and acceptance. Allow it to fill your entire being, knowing that this sense of self-compassion is always there for you to return to, like a comforting embrace. As you step back from the mirror, carry this feeling with you - a reminder of your worth, exactly as you are.

Echoes of Innocence

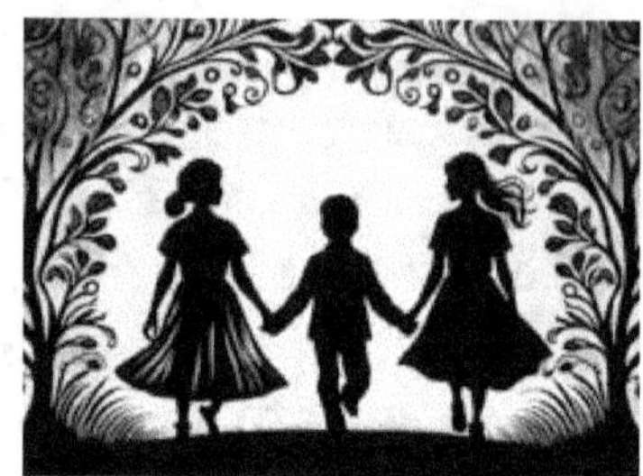

Transport yourself to a place familiar to you; a local park. One you might have visited many times, but today it feels different. This time, you're here with children—your own, or perhaps grandchildren, nieces, nephews, or young ones in your care. You notice their boundless energy, the way they run without hesitation, free and wild, their laughter bubbling over like a melody only they know. They're drawn to everything with equal fascination: a patch of wildflowers, an unusual stone, a puddle left by the morning rain, each discovery a new wonder in their world.

As they run and explore, you keep a mindful eye, ready to protect, yet allowing them the space to explore and discover on their own. Their innocence and joy are so pure and untouched, and you feel a pang of recognition. In their every gasp of awe, in their curious questions, and in their unselfconscious joy, you see a reflection of a part of yourself you had almost forgotten.

Memories begin to stir—moments when you, too, marveled at the world with wide-eyed wonder. When did that innocent joy slip into the background? When did the responsibilities and routines of adulthood bury this boundless, childlike spirit within you?

As you continue to watch, you feel a gentle urge to reconnect with that inner child, that part of you that was once equally enchanted with the world. You realize that this part of you—the one who once loved to play, to explore, to wonder—still exists. It may be hidden, softened by the years, but it's still there, waiting.

As the time comes to leave, you gather the children, feeling a sense of quiet resolve. You may be the adult now, full of responsibilities, but you don't have to lose the awe that once defined you. Perhaps you can carry that same lighthearted spirit forward, embracing wonder and curiosity wherever you find it. Today has been a reminder that the inner child, that playful, innocent part of you, is still alive and well, a spirit that can help you experience life with greater joy and compassion, not as a child, but with the wisdom of an open heart.

You leave the park with a subtle smile, knowing that your inner child is always there, ready to bring more wonder into each day.

XVII

Symphony at Sunrise

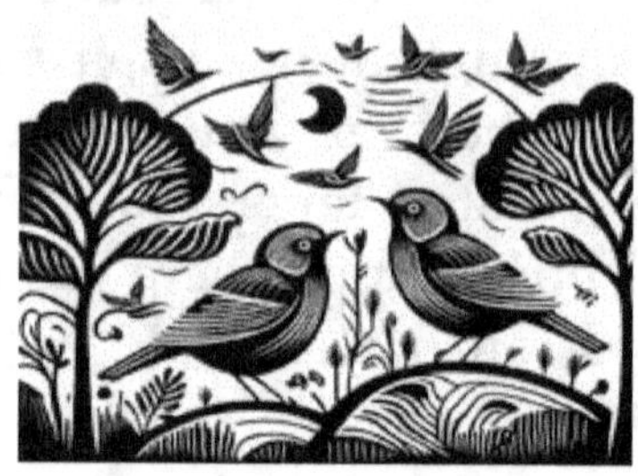

Imagine it's early morning, and you're drawn to a nearby woodland, eager to catch the sunrise. You step out into the fresh, cool air, and as you arrive at the edge of the trees, you feel a gentle mist lingering in the air, illuminated by the first hints of light. The grass is damp beneath your feet, inviting you to slip off your shoes. You step onto the soft, wet blades of grass, feeling each cool sensation grounding you to the earth.

You wander toward a small hill on the woodland's edge, a perfect vantage point for watching the dawn. You sit, settling in as the sun begins to break over the horizon, casting a warm, orange glow that softly touches your face. The warmth contrasts with the cool mist around you, wrapping you in a gentle embrace of light and stillness.

In the trees, birds are already alive with their morning songs. You close your eyes, letting the chorus grow, filling your senses with a symphony of life waking up. Each note rises and falls, echoing through the woodland, the perfect harmony of nature in full celebration of a new day.

Then, suddenly, there's a silence. You open your eyes and look around, noticing the absence of sound. Overhead, a hawk hovers, its form powerful and still against the sky. Its presence is striking and commanding, and you understand why the smaller birds have fallen silent. For a few minutes, this hunter moves in quiet control of the sky.

Then, as suddenly as it appeared, the hawk flies away, gliding into the distance. Gradually, the dawn chorus returns, the birds once more filling the air with their songs, even brighter and bolder than before.

As you sit there, watching and listening, it strikes you that life often has moments like this. Just as the hawk's presence temporarily stopped the birds, we all encounter things that disrupt our peace. Yet, like the dawn chorus, life's joys and natural rhythms return, just as they are meant to.

Let this remind you: when challenges or difficult people come your way, let them pass. They, like the hawk, are fleeting, unable to fully immerse in life's beauty. Remain steady in your joy, knowing that the peace and fullness of life will always come back.

Flight in Formation

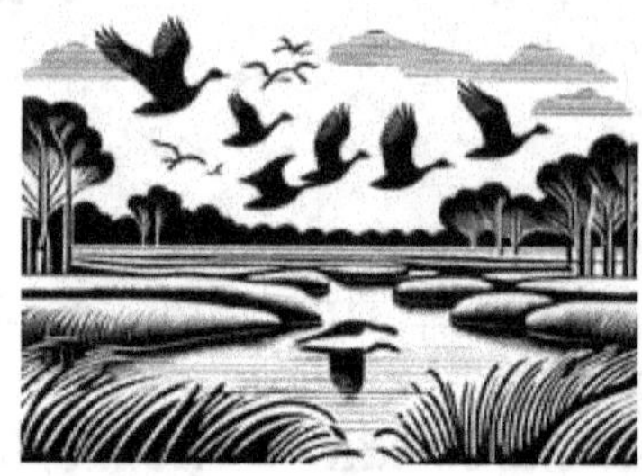

Let your mind wander to where you are walking along the flat, open marshes on a still morning, the kind that holds the first whispers of winter's arrival. There's a crispness to the air, a certain sharpness that brings everything into focus. The recent full moon has set a spring tide in motion, and you notice the water levels are a little higher, reflecting the silvery light that lingers even as dawn begins to creep across the sky. You're here for solitude, and you've found it—the only sound is your steady breath, accompanied by the soft squelch of earth beneath your feet.

The marsh stretches endlessly in every direction, and in this quiet, you feel deeply connected to the land, a part of the cycle that winter's touch has only just begun. But then, a sound breaks the silence—a distant honking that begins as a murmur and grows into a low, resonant symphony. You turn, scanning the horizon, and there, rising like a dark cloud in the distance, you see them: geese, hundreds upon hundreds, migrating from the colder reaches of the north, where winter has already laid its icy claim.

You lie back gently on the marsh, becoming one with the earth, so as not to startle the incoming flock. You watch as they approach, wave after wave, filling the sky above you. Ten, a hundred, a thousand—their numbers swell until the entire expanse is filled with them, each bird in perfect formation, honking in unison as they celebrate a journey spanning thousands of miles. The honking is deafening now, but you find it oddly calming, the sound vibrating through you, filling you with awe.

For a moment, they're so close it seems as though you could reach up and touch them. The geese, embodying strength and resilience, glide over you, shadows flickering across your face. They've crossed continents, defied elements, and braved the darkness to arrive here, to this exact moment. The marsh has become their sanctuary, just as it is yours.

Lying there, a profound respect washes over you. You're reminded of nature's raw intelligence, of the intricate cycles that carry creatures and elements alike. It's humbling, a reminder of your place in the grand design. As the geese disappear over the horizon, a deep gratitude settles within you. You carry this feeling with you, a quiet reverence for the spectacle you've witnessed, knowing it will remain with you throughout the day, a gift from nature herself.

XIX

Strings in Harmony

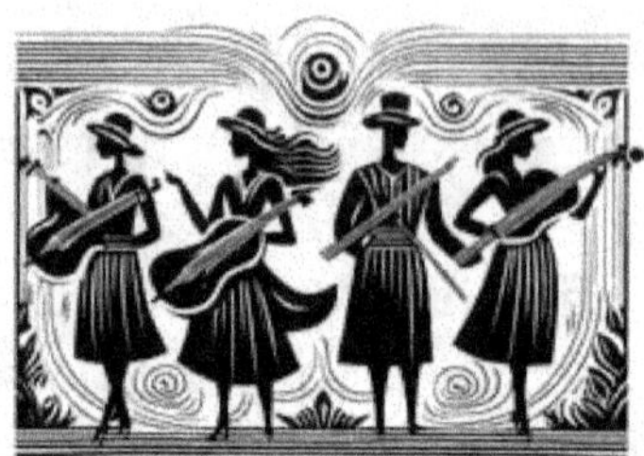

Close your eyes and place the headphones over your ears, allowing the sounds of the string quartet to fill your mind. The first notes flow gently, like ripples across a calm lake, as the violins, viola, and cello begin their delicate dance. Each sound feels rich and layered, as if it's reaching out to you across time, telling a story crafted hundreds of years ago.

The music moves with an effortless grace, and you can sense the composer's genius woven into every measure. This piece was written in a time long past by a person with rare, extraordinary talent - someone who poured their heart and mind into each note, intending only that others might find joy in hearing it. And yet, they could never have imagined their music would one day reach listeners through modern technology, on a device like the one you hold.

Your thoughts shift to the musicians performing this piece. Their skill is masterful, honed over countless hours of practice and dedication. You wonder about each one - who they are, whether they're still with us, or if they're playing this somewhere far away, blissfully unaware of how their talent is reaching you right now. These performers are at the height of their craft, fully immersed in their art, even though they may never know exactly who will be touched by it.

Then, you think of the instruments themselves. The violins, the cello, the viola; all were crafted by hands that knew wood, sound, and patience in a way few do. Each instrument reflects the care and expertise of someone who understood how to shape wood and strings into vessels of harmony. Their skill lives on, even without them knowing who might enjoy the fruits of their labor.

A sense of gratitude and awe fills you. You realize how many skilled and dedicated people came together, across generations, to create this one experience for you. They weren't working just for recognition or reward but out of passion and a desire to share beauty, regardless of who might be listening. You feel a deep appreciation for this invisible chain of artists and craftspeople whose efforts culminate in this moment, allowing you to experience their art. And though you can't thank them directly, you feel that your enjoyment honors their dedication.

Take a breath, letting that feeling of gratitude settle within you. You are connected to these creators through their work, a part of something timeless and beautiful.

XX

Through the Amber

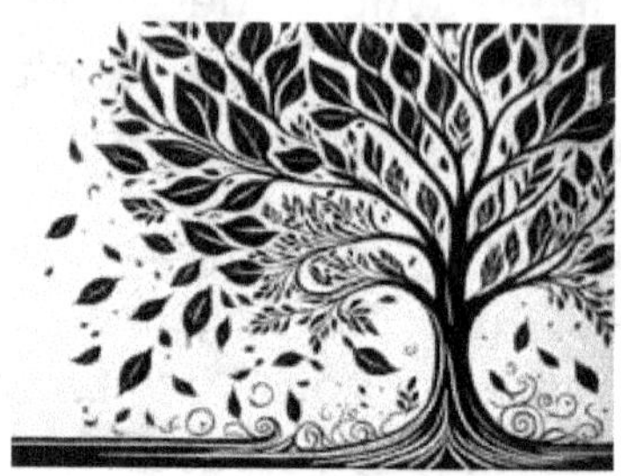

You walk slowly through an ancient woodland on a golden autumn evening, each step softly crunching leaves that lay scattered across the trail. Above you, branches of towering oaks and elegant beeches stretch out, their limbs still bearing patches of brilliant color. Shades of fiery red, deep orange, and luminous gold are illuminated by the sun's warm glow, intensifying the leaves' hues until they seem almost otherworldly in their beauty. A gentle breeze weaves through, and as it does, leaves drift lazily to the ground, swirling gracefully in the amber light.

As you walk further, you come upon a thick, inviting bed of leaves —so deep and rich that it seems to cushion the forest floor with a natural warmth. Without a second thought, you step off the path and let yourself sink onto the pile. The leaves cradle you, softening your landing, their earthy scent rising as they press gently beneath you, absorbing the weight as if they've been waiting to offer this comfort. It's quiet here; even your breath seems to soften, blending with the forest sounds.

You lie back, watching the leaves above shift in the breeze, a few drifting down, twirling as they fall, each leaf floating in its own gentle descent. It's a reminder of the cycle of life, these leaves that once flourished with green vitality, now finding rest upon the earth. Somehow, the stillness of this autumn scene stirs a quiet contemplation within you. You feel the changing of the seasons as a reflection of your own journey, each fallen leaf a symbol of life's inevitable cycles.

The sun sinks lower, its light softening as it brushes through the branches, casting long, tender shadows that blend with the gathering dusk. You find yourself pondering these shifts, the way life gives way to rest, and how from that rest, life is renewed again. There is a beauty, even a reassurance, in this quiet letting go, and a soft realization rises within you: just as the forest knows when to shed and renew, so does the journey of your own life, enriched by every experience.

In this moment, surrounded by the tender embrace of nature, you feel deeply alive, touched by an inexplicable sense of peace. The world feels expansive, endless even, and somehow, lying here, you sense the grace in the passing of time. It all feels sacred, each moment a gift that, like the leaves, falls gently but leaves its mark on the heart.

XXI

Serenity in the Cove

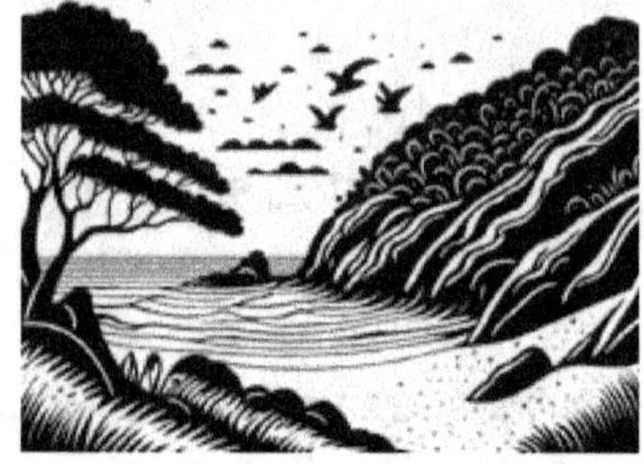

Following the path through the short grass dotted with daisies & buttercups, the warmth of a summer morning envelops you, your bare feet sensing the slight prickle of the grass on their soles. Reaching the top of ancient wooden stairs, you slowly descend, feeling the gritty texture of the sand drifted onto the steps from the dunes. Your hand glides down the handrail worn smooth by many generations of beachgoers as you reach the shore and walk over the almost unbearably hot sand.

Relief washes over you as you feel the cooler wet sand underfoot, entering the shallow water of the cove. The sea is calm, barely lapping at the beach, sunbeams dancing on the surface like diamonds while ripples reflect on the sand beneath. Sensations envelop you - the heat of the sun on your face, the taste of salt on your lips, and the echo of seagulls' cries in your ears.

Deeper into the water, you duck below the surface and emerge to float on your back. Submerged, all previous sounds are silenced, replaced only by the beat of your heart and the pulse of the waves against the shore. Eventually, a matching rhythm settles, and you feel at one with nature. Swimming back to the shore, you enjoy the flex and pull of your muscles against the water, feeling strong as you return to the beach, finding a spot to lie down and doze in the sunshine, letting the heat from the sun dry your clothing.

As the sounds of seabirds are joined by the laughter of children and the low hum of conversation, the realisation dawns that the cove is no longer yours alone. Rising to your feet, you ascend the worn steps, leaving behind the tranquil sanctuary of the cove, you carry with you the memory of the harmony you found in nature's embrace.

In this journey, you discovered a profound truth: that moments of serenity are not possessions to be clung to, but gifts to be shared. The laughter of children and the chatter of companions remind you that amidst the solitude of self-discovery, there is also joy in the shared experience of existence. Each step upward symbolizes the return to the bustling world beyond, where connections with others enrich the tapestry of life. And as you reach the top, you realize that the tranquillity you sought below is not lost, but rather, it resides within you, ready to be summoned whenever you seek solace amidst the chaos of existence.

Guardians of Time

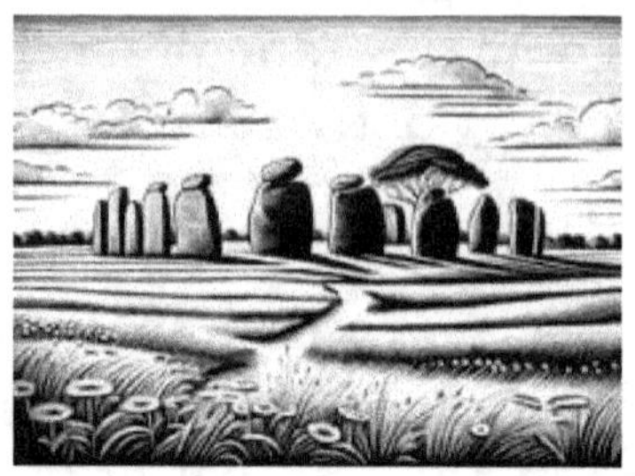

Picture yourself arriving at an ancient stone circle on a still, misty morning. The stones rise from the ground like sentries, partially hidden by the fog. You walk slowly into the heart of the circle, feeling the weight of its silence, as if it's holding a memory too vast to share all at once. The air feels thick with anticipation, as though it's waiting for you to settle in and become still.

You take your seat at the center, lowering yourself to the earth, allowing your body to find comfort against the cool, damp ground. Closing your eyes, you breathe deeply, letting each exhale carry away any lingering thoughts. You begin to tune in to the subtle sounds of the morning—the occasional bird call, the faint rustle of mist-laden grass, and the gentle hum of presence in the air around you. Here, you're enclosed in solitude, embraced by a circle that has witnessed millennia.

As you sink further into stillness, you open your eyes to see the stones more clearly. Rising tall and steadfast, they seem timeless, as if they've always been here, waiting through ages of sun and storm, watching humanity come and go. These stones, partially veiled by the mist, look like ancient guardians, their edges softened, yet strong, casting a feeling of permanence that feels almost impossible. You're left to wonder why they were placed here, the purpose they served, and the hands that shaped and lifted them.

Were they markers of a journey, guiding those who came before? A place to celebrate, honor, or simply witness the cycles of the sun and stars? Perhaps they held the whispers of a people who, like you, came searching for answers. You'll never know, but the mystery feels strangely comforting, like an invitation to embrace the unknown.

You begin to feel a presence—a subtle energy all around you, a quiet sense of belonging in this ancient space. You imagine someone, many thousands of years ago, sitting just as you are now, searching for wisdom, for insight, for a way to feel connected to something greater. You can almost sense them, their breath matching yours, their heartbeat echoing across time.

In that moment, you feel the boundary between past and present fade. It dawns on you that the search for meaning, for connection, is something that transcends time. The same wonder, the same yearning lives within you as it did within them. You realize that, like the builders of this circle, you're part of a lineage of seekers, all drawn to something that can't be seen but only felt, something eternal and sacred.

Viewing Platform

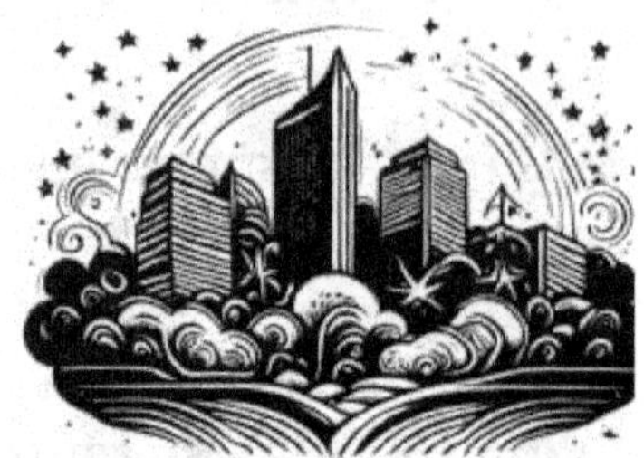

Where might your breath take you today? See yourself stepping into a sleek, mirrored elevator in the towering heart of a city that never quite sleeps. You press the button for the topmost floor of a renowned skyscraper - perhaps an iconic tower with breathtaking views. It's late, and the building is closing soon, so you're likely to be one of the last visitors. As the elevator glides upwards, the soft hum and occasional shudder are all you hear. You feel your ears pop with the ascent, a gentle reminder of the height you're reaching. With each floor that passes, you anticipate what lies above, the city shrinking beneath you.

At last, the doors slide open, and you step out onto the observation platform, the final visitor of the night. A brisk, cold wind greets you immediately, whipping through the wire mesh surrounding the platform. The city lights stretch in every direction, a mesmerizing sea of glimmers. Rows of streetlamps carve out avenues; headlights snake along unseen highways; office towers, still lit up, pulse with the quiet hum of night workers. There's an organized chaos to it all - a delicate web of countless lives, each engaged in its own rhythm. Yet, here, standing above it all, you are utterly alone in silence.

You walk to the edge and look out, struck by the vastness and beauty of the lights that surround you. It's an overwhelming realization that you're part of this city right now, but in a fleeting way - an unnoticed figure in the thousands of lives below, each life unaware of yours, and you unaware of theirs. At this moment, none of them know you're here, that you've reached this peculiar peak. You're the highest person in the city, perched atop a metropolis teeming with lives and stories, some just waking to the night and others winding down. A tiny detail to you, but somehow it feels profound, even humorous—a small, secret victory in a sea of people who will never know you were here.

The experience makes you wonder about connection and solitude, about being a part of something grand yet remaining separate. It's humbling, this realization that you're one star in a galaxy of human existence - small yet brilliant in your own right. You breathe in the cold, high air, feeling connected to the city below but also, strangely, above it. And as you stand there, you feel a quiet acceptance of being just one among many - an invisible presence in a world so busy with itself. For now, that feels freeing. You watch the lights blink below, breathe in one last, deep breath, and decide that sometimes, simply being is enough.

XXIV

Savasana I

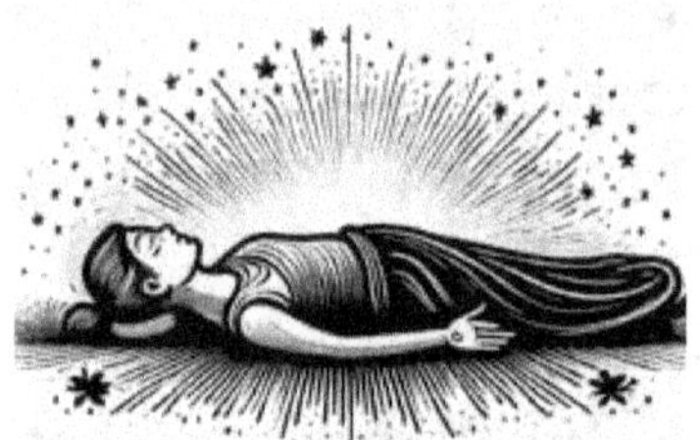

Begin by lying comfortably on your mat, adjusting your position until you feel completely at ease. Allow your legs to extend naturally, letting your feet fall open to the sides. Rest your arms gently at your sides, with your palms facing upward, ready to receive calm and relaxation. Close your eyes and take a slow, deep breath, feeling your body soften as you exhale.

With each breath, let your body become heavier, feeling yourself gently sinking, melting into the support of the mat. Imagine that each exhale lets you release any last bit of tension, allowing gravity to cradle and support you fully.

Now, visualize a gentle, soothing wave beginning at the very tips of your toes. This wave, calm and warm, slowly rises over your feet, bringing a sense of deep relaxation as it moves up to your ankles. Feel it washing over each toe, releasing any tightness, softening your feet completely. With every exhale, feel this wave washing stress away.

The wave of calm rises to your calves, flowing like warm water, gently dissolving any tension in each muscle, easing your legs into peaceful rest. It continues up, softly wrapping around your knees and then reaching your thighs, spreading that feeling of calm and comfort deep into your muscles. Let each breath help you sink even deeper into stillness.

As the wave reaches your hips, allow it to flow through your lower back and abdomen, gently releasing any held tension. Imagine this calming wave soothing your spine, bringing ease and lightness with every breath.

Now, the wave rises to your chest, soothing your heart, slowing your breath to a gentle, natural rhythm. Feel the wave's warmth move up to your shoulders, softening them, allowing them to release any weight you might be carrying. Sense your entire torso melting into relaxation, held securely by the mat.

This wave flows from your shoulders, drifting slowly down each arm. It travels through your upper arms, easing your elbows, your forearms, and wrists. As it reaches your fingertips, you feel the last traces of tension releasing, slipping away, leaving only peace.

Finally, the wave moves up through your neck, easing away any tightness, softening your throat. It rises to your face, smoothing your jaw, releasing your cheeks, softening your eyes, and finally reaching the very top of your head. Feel your entire body now resting in perfect peace, held in a state of calm and ease.

Allow yourself to stay here, held by the mat, your body and mind completely relaxed, each part of you resting in stillness and calm. There's nothing you need to do but breathe gently, allowing yourself to simply be, fully at peace, deeply relaxed.

XXV

Grace in Motion

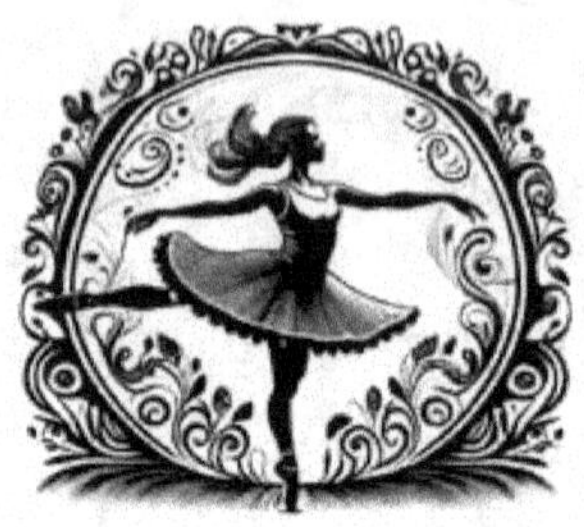

Have you ever wanted to be a dancer? Well, picture yourself standing in the middle of a grand, empty stage, bathed in soft, warm light. You're dressed in elegant ballet attire, a delicate costume that moves like silk against your skin. There's a faint murmur in the audience, but it's distant, barely reaching your ears. What fills you is the music—a gentle melody at first, a graceful tune that flows around you and seems to seep into your bones. It's as though you and the music are one, your body responding without hesitation, instinctively attuned to the rhythm.

As you take your first steps, you glide into a *plié*, gently bending your knees as your arms float upward, hands shaping delicately in time with the melody. Without a thought, you sweep into an *arabesque*, one leg extending behind you, arms reaching forward with poise, as if to pull you towards the music itself. You feel your body elongate, your movements graceful, and you are both grounded and free, gliding across the stage as if weightless.

The music builds, and so does your confidence. You attempt a *pirouette*, turning on the tips of your toes, spinning in perfect harmony with the music. The world blurs around you as you twirl, your arms held just so, and the sensation is exhilarating. The music quickens, and without hesitation, you leap into a *grand jeté*, soaring through the air, suspended in perfect flight before landing with a soft, almost inaudible touch.

Your heart races as the music swells, and you let it carry you further. Your body begins to move with more daring, more freedom—executing a *fouetté en tournant*, one leg extended in a graceful arc as you spin in place, your body a living expression of the music's crescendo. You feel alive, powerful, each turn and leap filling you with a newfound confidence.

The melody reaches its peak, and with every ounce of energy, you prepare for a final, awe-inspiring move—a *grand fouetté*. You pivot, your leg whipping in a high, perfect arc, your body turning gracefully as the motion carries you across the stage. It feels like magic, an impossible beauty made real in this single, breathtaking moment.

Finally, as the music fades, you come to a poised halt, arms extended and head lifted toward the lights, which now shine brightly upon you, illuminating your every move. For a moment, there is silence. Then, like a wave, you hear the applause, the sound of cheers and joy filling the theater, echoing in your ears. An unseen audience is standing in rapture, celebrating this dance, this perfect connection between you and the music.

And as you stand there, breathless but alive with exhilaration, you feel a quiet, profound joy, knowing that in this moment, you have danced not just for others, but for yourself.

XXVI

Crisp Air, Clean Mind

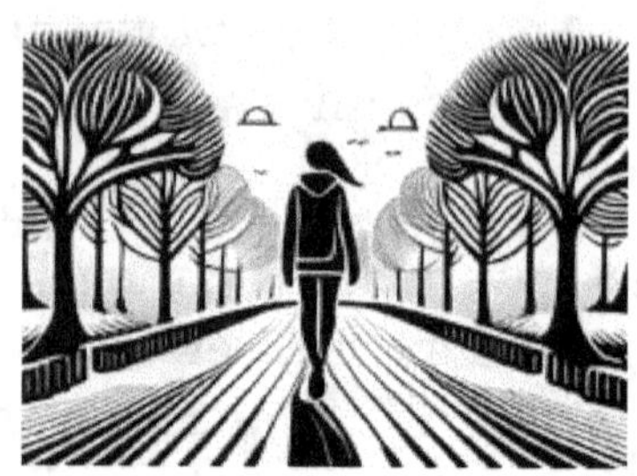

L et your mind wander and imagine yourself on a peaceful country path, surrounded by the gentle beauty of nature. It's a crisp morning, the sun low in the sky, casting a soft golden light that catches on the dew resting along the grass and leaves. The air is fresh, filling your lungs with the quiet strength of the countryside. Birds are singing softly, their calls weaving in and out of the gentle rustle of trees in the light breeze. You feel the solid earth beneath your feet, your steps soft on the worn path.

As you walk, breathing in the calmness of this place, you hear the distant hum of a car approaching. Slowly, you step off the path, onto the soft grass, giving space for it to pass. As it draws closer, you notice it's a sleek, luxury car, polished and glinting in the morning sun. Behind the wheel, the driver sits with an air of importance, dressed sharply, and his wrist catches the light; a sleek, shining watch gleaming. A cigar rests between his fingers, leaving a faint trace of smoke that mingles with the morning air.

The car slows briefly as it comes near, and you lift your hand, a simple wave, acknowledging the presence of a fellow traveler. But his gaze stays straight ahead, his expression set and determined, as though he's already elsewhere, mind racing toward a destination, a deal, or a deadline that seems more important than this moment. For a second, you wonder if he even saw you or if he's simply too absorbed in his own world, each minute accounted for, each action meticulously planned.

The car speeds off, its roar fading into the distance, leaving you in the quiet again. You return to the path, feeling the soft morning breeze on your skin and noticing how clear and fresh the air feels. You breathe deeply, enjoying the simple freedom of this stroll, where there's no rush, no place you must be. You pause to watch the clouds drift lazily across the sky, the sun now just a bit higher, warming your face.

And as you continue walking, a thought settles into your mind: there are different kinds of wealth. One kind may be counted in material luxuries, the gleam of a car, the shine of a watch. But another kind, perhaps less obvious, is found here; in the space to take in the beauty around you, the freedom to walk at your own pace, to greet the world openly, with ease.

In this stillness, you feel a quiet richness, a wealth of simplicity and peace that belongs to you alone. And perhaps, in this moment, you realize that wealth can take many forms, and true abundance is in seeing, feeling, and breathing it all in, here, now.

Halls of Wonder

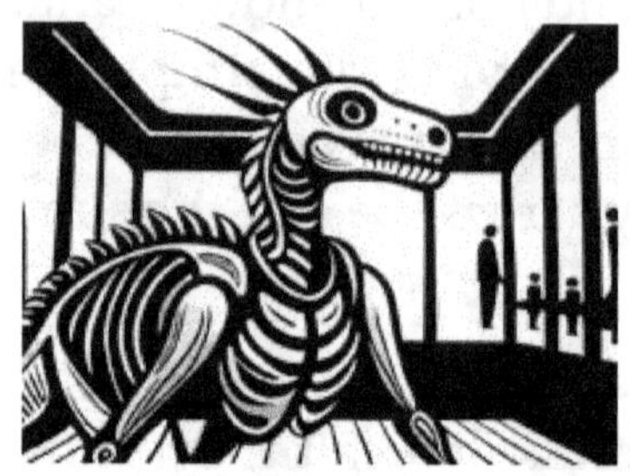

It begins with a single step into an old-fashioned museum. The kind where the air feels thick with dust and mystery, where the light filtering through tall, narrow windows is dim and golden, casting long shadows over the polished floors. There's an almost eerie silence, save for the soft echoes of your footsteps. This museum, a grand relic from another time, stands frozen with a certain solemnity, its high vaulted ceilings and faded wallpaper whispering stories of ages past. The carved, wooden door creaks shut behind you, sealing you into this sanctuary of ancient human achievements.

The rooms are lined with cabinets of curiosities from across the world. You pass shelves of meticulously preserved artifacts: African masks with carved, watchful eyes; delicate flint tools, sharp-edged and chipped by hands long gone; towering dinosaur skeletons, jaws forever frozen in silent roars, and majestic Egyptian mummies, wrapped in linen, their expressions stoic and otherworldly. The stuffed animals and birds seem to look back at you, their glass eyes glinting in the dim light. Everything here is a testament to the ingenuity of human curiosity, a universal desire to capture the essence of life, of time, and the natural world. Each piece is a reminder of the lengths to which we've gone to understand our surroundings, to document, preserve, and marvel at the world's vast beauty.

As you wander deeper, you begin to sense that no single culture holds claim to superiority here. Instead, this vast collection stands as a mosaic of human endeavor. Each culture represented — from the flint-knapping societies to the skilled carvers of African art and the ancient Egyptian morticians — reveals a shared curiosity, a drive to seek answers, and an appreciation for the beauty that surrounds us. It becomes clear that, across millennia and continents, humankind has continually striven to preserve knowledge, to make sense of existence, and to contribute a unique thread to the fabric of our collective history.

As you make your way back toward the entrance, the creak of a door signals the arrival of a group of schoolchildren. Their excited chatter and quick footsteps echo down the hall, momentarily breaking the museum's quiet spell. A slight smile comes to your face as you step aside, grateful for the solitude you've had but aware that these children, with their eager, fresh eyes, are now being given their own chance to marvel, question, and connect with these artifacts. They are part of the continuum, future custodians of knowledge and curiosity. As they explore this treasure trove of human history, you realize they will one day pass these lessons forward to the next generation, continuing the cycle that has bound humans together through ages.

With one last look at the grandeur of the museum, you step back into the world outside, carrying a sense of connection not just to the past, but to the future as well.

Remembrance

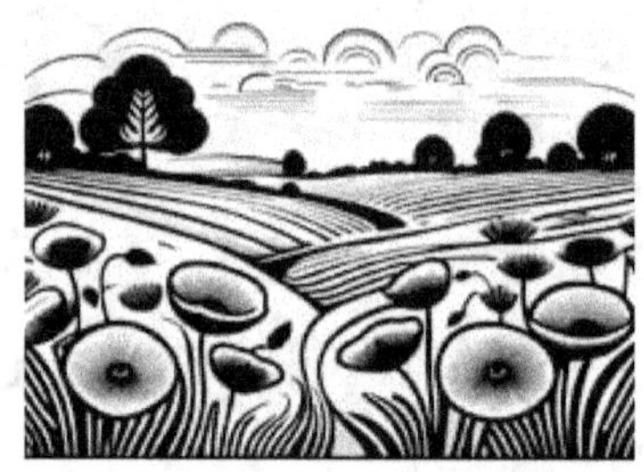

See yourself standing in a wide, open field. Golden autumn grasses stretch out all around you, swaying with a gentle rhythm as a soft breeze moves through them, creating a whisper that seems to echo through the vast space. You take a slow, grounding breath, feeling yourself becoming part of this open landscape, the horizon stretching as far as the eye can see.

Ahead, you notice a pathway lined with bright red poppies. Their petals are delicate yet vivid, catching the morning light like small flames dotting the earth. Slowly, you begin walking along this path, feeling each step connect you more deeply with the solid earth beneath. The soil feels firm and reassuring underfoot, each step grounding you in the present moment.

As you walk, you notice smooth stones laid thoughtfully along the way. They sit quietly, each one seemingly bearing the weight of countless memories, silent witnesses to the lives that have passed. These stones carry stories—stories of courage, resilience, and hope, reminders of those who faced their own challenges with quiet strength.

Pause here for a moment. Allow yourself to connect to the spirit of these lives, to the strength and courage of those who came before you. Let a wave of gratitude rise within you, honoring those who have touched this world with their presence. The stones feel timeless and wise, their strength enduring like the memory of those who have faced life's trials with open hearts and enduring spirits.

As you take in the landscape, the red poppies continue to sway gently in the breeze. They stand as symbols of hope and resilience, a reminder of the beauty that persists even in times of difficulty. Notice how their vibrant color contrasts against the earth, a celebration of life, a reminder of courage.

Gently place your hands over your heart, letting a feeling of gratitude settle within. Feel a deep, steady connection to all that has come before you, all the love and resilience that has paved the way for you to stand here today. Take a deep breath, inhaling this sense of peace, letting it fill you completely.

Now, as you exhale, release any tension, any worry or heaviness. With each exhale, feel yourself letting go, emptying what you no longer need. Let your heart feel light, as though each breath frees you, connecting you to a sense of calm and timeless strength.

In this moment, feel that you are part of an unbroken chain, connected to the lives that have shaped this world. With every beat of your heart, know that you carry forward the courage and compassion of those who came before, and that your own journey is woven into the same tapestry of life and resilience.

Take one more deep breath, feeling this sense of connection and strength expanding within you. Let your heart be filled with gratitude, carrying this calm and enduring energy forward into the rest of your day, knowing that you, too, are a part of this shared story of life.

XXIX

Petals of Time

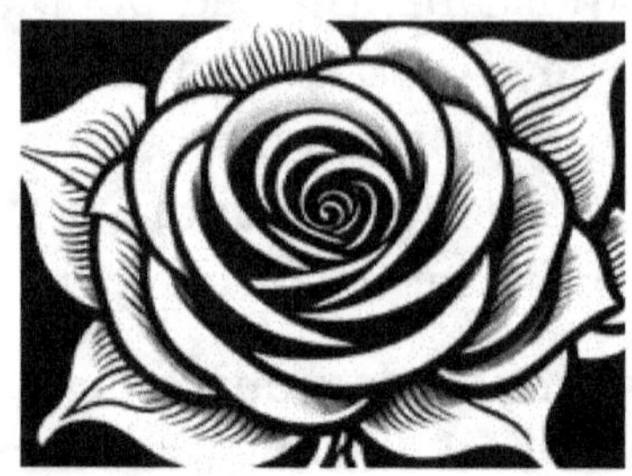

Imagine you are sitting alone in a quiet, undisturbed space, holding a single, radiant rose in your hands. You've chosen this time to be still, to simply focus on this rose, to be entirely present with its beauty. Bringing it closer to your face, you admire how the deep red petals have unfurled into a perfect, layered spiral. Each petal has opened in delicate circles, like nature's own artwork, radiating outward to form a complete, intricate bloom.

As you gaze at it, you notice the richness of its color—a deep, velvet red that seems almost alive, pulsing with vitality. You turn the flower gently on its stem, studying the soft gradients of red, noticing how the petals near the edges have relaxed outward, while those nearer the center remain tucked, revealing hints of the flower's core. It feels like a miracle, this moment of perfect form. Each petal is unique yet seamlessly part of the whole.

Leaning in, you inhale the rose's fragrance—a scent that feels both earthy and sweet, delicate yet potent, like the promise of life itself. It's a scent so subtle, so enchanting, you close your eyes just to absorb it fully. The faint tickling of tiny stamens crowned with hints of golden pollen brushes your nose, grounding you in the physical world even as your mind drifts, enchanted by the flower's timeless beauty.

For a while, you are completely immersed, as if the outside world has disappeared. But then, as you continue to watch, you notice a subtle change. The outer petals seem to lose a little of their vibrancy, the edges curling inward. Slowly, the once-radiant red begins to fade to a softer, muted shade. You watch as the petals begin to dry, their silky texture transforming into something fragile, brittle. The rose, in your hands, ages before your eyes.

The scent, too, begins to fade, leaving only a trace of its former sweetness. You witness the slow withering of this bloom, once so full of life, now slumping as its petals loosen, some drifting downward. In a moment, it is no longer the same vibrant rose that filled you with awe. It is something different now—a quieter beauty, a reminder of what once was.

And as you sit with this transformation, you realize that the life of this rose mirrors our own journey. Like the rose, we blossom in vitality, radiating our own colors, until time gently pulls us toward our own softening, fading. There is a bittersweet beauty in this, a quiet inevitability. And yet, just as with the rose, our time in bloom is precious, filled with meaning and joy.

Reflecting on this, you don't feel sadness for the rose's passing. Instead, you feel a deep gratitude for having witnessed it, for the brief but beautiful moment it gave to the world. You understand that, like all of us, it was here to be celebrated and remembered not for its end, but for the life it held within its petals, the gift it shared at its peak.

XXX

Song of a Thrush

With your eyes closed take a deep breath, feeling the air move through you, as gentle as a whisper. In your mind's eye, you find yourself in a lush, green meadow bordered by a dense forest. The golden light of dawn filters through the trees, casting a soft glow over the grasses swaying in the breeze. The air is alive with the hum of life; the rustling of leaves, the distant babble of a brook, and the faint, melodic call of a bird.

You step forward, drawn to the sound, each note weaving through the air like threads of sunlight. Your feet follow a well-worn path through the meadow and into the forest beyond. Here, the trees form a natural cathedral, their branches arching overhead to create a sanctuary of calm and peace. You feel sheltered, embraced by the warm stillness, with only the occasional flutter of wings breaking the quiet.

As you wander deeper, the song grows clearer; a rich, fluid melody, full of emotion and strength. The source of the sound reveals itself: a song thrush perched on a low-hanging branch, its feathers a mix of tawny brown and speckled white, glowing in the soft light. Its throat swells with each note, and you feel its song reach into the depths of your soul, stirring something deep within.

The bird looks directly at you, tilting its head as if inviting you to listen more closely. Its song seems to carry a message; not in words, but in feeling. It is a song of resilience and courage, of embracing your unique voice and letting it be heard.

The thrush flutters down to a nearby rock, and without hesitation, it begins to sing again. You watch in awe as the sound ripples through the air, filling the forest with a quiet, undeniable power. Something stirs within you; a memory of times when you held back your words, when fear or doubt made you silent.

You feel the thrush's melody calling to you, encouraging you to let go of that hesitation. You imagine your voice as strong and clear as the bird's song, flowing freely like water from a spring. You take a deep breath, and as you exhale, you feel a shift within—like a lock clicking open or a river breaking free of its dam.

The thrush pauses, looking at you once more, as if to say, *Now it's your turn.* You feel the weight of the moment, not as pressure, but as an invitation. You place a hand on your throat, feeling the vibration of your breath, imagining the power of your words waiting to be released.

When you are ready, you give a silent nod to the bird. Its wings spread wide, and it takes to the sky, circling once before vanishing into the canopy above. Its song lingers in the air, echoing softly, as if it has left a part of itself with you.

You turn back along the path, feeling lighter, freer, and filled with a quiet determination to let your voice be heard. The melody of the thrush remains with you, a reminder of the power and beauty of finding your own song.

XXXI

Ripples of a Pond

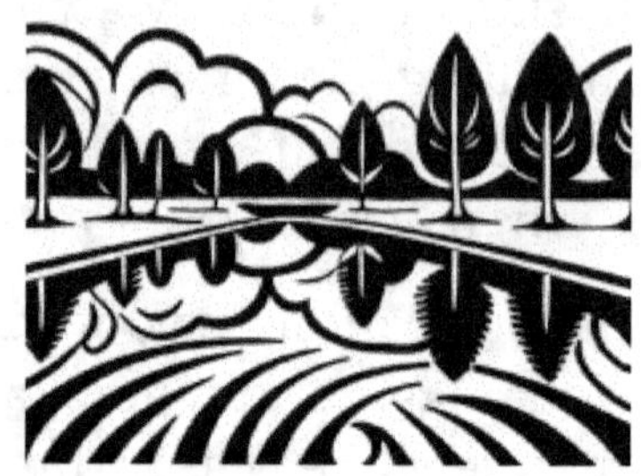

Take a moment to settle your breath as we begin and picture yourself at the edge of a large still pond on an early morning. You've come here because sleep didn't come easily last night, your mind swirling with thoughts and concerns that linger in the early light. The air around you is calm and misty, with a soft orange glow from the sun rising just above the horizon, casting warm light over everything in sight.

The pond before you is perfectly still, mirroring the misty sky and the orange sun. You begin to walk slowly along the edge, each step mindful, hearing only the soft crunch of earth beneath your feet. With each step, you admire the peacefulness of the pond's surface, wondering if your own mind could reflect this stillness. You find yourself drawn into a rhythm of breathing, in sync with the stillness surrounding you, feeling your own restlessness beginning to quiet.

Through the haze of morning mist, you notice a figure walking toward you. An elderly man in an orange robe, with a shaved head and gentle smile, approaches you. As he reaches you, he places his hands together in greeting, quietly saying, "Namaste." His eyes hold a warmth that feels both welcoming and wise, as though he's familiar with the troubles you've carried into the day. Somehow, he seems to know that sleep eluded you, and as he looks at you, he murmurs, "You've come here with a busy mind."

The simplicity of his words takes you by surprise, and you feel seen in a way that is both unsettling and comforting. Without waiting for you to respond, he gently bends down and picks up a small pebble from the ground. Turning to the pond, he holds it up, allowing you to focus on its shape and weight, and then, in one swift motion, he tosses it into the center of the water.

You watch as the pebble strikes the pond's surface, creating concentric ripples that spread out in widening circles. As the ripples move farther from the center, they begin to slow, their energy eventually fading until the pond becomes mirror-still once more.

"These ripples," the man says softly, "are like your thoughts and emotions. Each one arises, moves outward, and eventually fades back into calm. No matter how restless, they always return to stillness."

You stand quietly, absorbing his words, as the last ripple fades completely and the pond is again perfectly still. A sense of calm washes over you, and without realizing it, you feel your own thoughts beginning to settle, like the ripples becoming quiet. The man simply smiles at you, his gaze warm and knowing, as if he already senses the quiet within you.

As you turn to thank him, you realize he is gone, as silently as he appeared, leaving you alone at the water's edge. Gazing into the still pond, you sense that you, too, can release the ripples of your mind, allowing them to fade and return to a place of inner calm whenever they arise. With this newfound peace, you breathe deeply, feeling lighter, knowing that, like the pond, you can find stillness within yourself, letting each thought and emotion drift into calm.

XXXII

Sea Wanderer

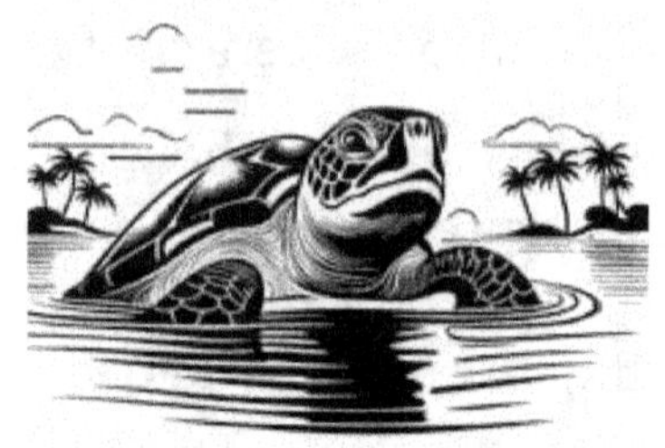

Imagine yourself on a tropical beach, where the sand is warm and golden beneath you, like fine grains of sunlight scattered across the shore. The sea stretches out in shades of turquoise and blue, its gentle waves rolling in soft whispers, brushing up against the sand before retreating in rhythmic peace. Tall palm trees sway behind you, their fronds casting long shadows in the warm, golden glow of the late afternoon. The air is filled with the faint scent of salt and the occasional cry of seabirds soaring overhead.

You settle into a meditative posture, feeling the soft sand molding beneath you. You take a deep breath, absorbing the sounds, the warmth, and the slow, soothing pulse of the ocean. You close your eyes, drifting into a space where it's just you, the earth, and the endless sea.

Suddenly, a splash breaks your focus, subtle yet close enough to draw your attention. Opening your eyes, you glance out toward the water. At first, you see only the smooth surface of the waves, but then you spot it—a head poking up from the water. For a moment, you think it might be a seal, but as you focus, you realize it's something even rarer. It's a sea turtle, its dark eyes and ancient face peeking above the waterline, observing you with a calm curiosity.

A wave of joy washes over you. Sea turtles have become a rare sight here, and knowing you've spent countless hours volunteering to protect them makes this encounter feel special, like a reward for years of quiet work. Usually, turtles are cautious and shy, and this one's boldness strikes you as unusual.

But then, something even stranger happens. Rather than disappearing back into the ocean, the turtle paddles closer, moving steadily toward the shore until it's only a few feet from the beach. Its large shell breaks the surface, glistening in the sunlight, and you can see its flippers paddling gracefully below. Then, to your astonishment, it begins to walk—slowly, deliberately—out of the water.

The turtle's flippers dig into the sand, pulling its large body forward with surprising ease, leaving deep tracks behind it. It waddles up to you, stopping just a few feet away. Its ancient, dark eyes meet yours, and you feel an undeniable connection. The turtle's eyes are deep, wise, and warm, reflecting the age and mystery of the ocean. In its gaze, you see a quiet intelligence, a calm awareness that feels almost otherworldly.

For a long moment, you simply look at each other, and then it dawns on you: this turtle recognizes you. Over the years, you've saved countless baby turtles, guiding them safely into the sea, out of reach of hungry seagulls and other predators. You can't possibly remember each tiny life you've helped along its journey, but somehow, this one remembers you.

The turtle blinks slowly, almost as if nodding, and in that gaze, you understand. This is a thank you—simple, profound, and wordless. You never expected gratitude for the work you've done, but this feels like the most precious gift you could receive. It's a moment beyond words, a rare acknowledgment of kindness given and kindness received, from one life to another. After a time, the turtle lowers its head and turns back toward the ocean, leaving you with a sense of wonder and fulfillment that will remain long after it disappears back beneath the waves.

XXXIII

Boundless Heights

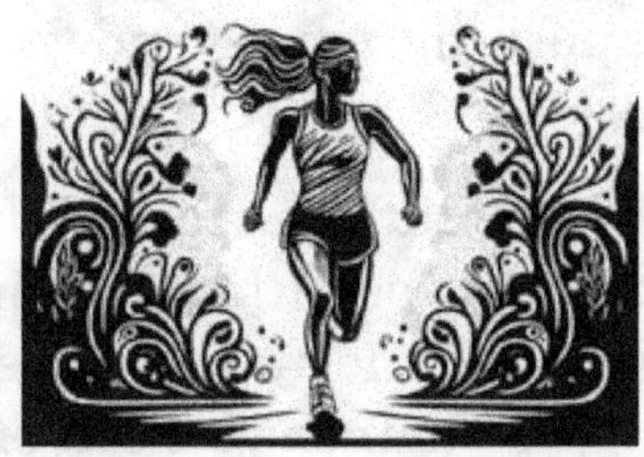

You are at the base of a towering mountain, its jagged peaks cutting through a vast, clear sky. Dressed in your running gear, you stretch your legs, feeling each muscle as it readies for action. The air is pristine, crisp and exhilarating, with a hint of pine and earth from the trails winding up the mountainside. You take a deep breath, savoring that fresh alpine scent, and place your headphones over your ears, catching the subtle buzz of anticipation.

The track begins softly; a steady beat, gaining intensity. You feel the bass in your chest, syncing with your own heartbeat, and you rock back and forth in place, muscles tightening, ready to explode into motion. Then, as if on cue, the beat kicks in, a driving rhythm that surges through you. Your body responds instantly, and you're off, legs powering forward with an effortless strength, heart pounding in time to the music.

As you race uphill, your stride feels light, natural. There's an exhilarating sense of freedom in every step. Usually, your muscles would be protesting by now, but today is different. Your legs, your lungs, every fiber of your body is tuned to this moment, a perfect symphony of movement and music. You feel like you could fly up the mountain. The slope is steep, but you're moving fast, bounding over rocks and uneven ground with ease. You can feel the rush of wind against your face, cool and refreshing, and your breathing stays steady, strong, in perfect sync with your pace.

The trail flattens, and you let yourself push harder, almost sprinting along the narrow, winding path. Your senses sharpen; you hear the crunch of gravel underfoot, the rhythmic pulse of your breath, the distant call of a bird. Each beat of the music drives you faster, every note pushing you beyond your limits. It's as if the mountain is your playground, and you're fully in your element.

The climb steepens again, but the energy pulsing through your veins keeps you going. You bend low, leaning into the incline, each step powerful, focused. The music crescendos, and suddenly, without even thinking, you launch yourself off a rock, executing a perfect front somersault mid-air. Time seems to slow as you twist, the world blurring, then snapping back into focus as you land, steady and exhilarated. The music eases into a slower, deeper beat, as if rewarding your perfect move.

As you near the summit, the path fades, rocks and boulders now scattered before you. It doesn't matter; you're ready for anything. You leap from rock to rock, the rhythm of the music guiding your every movement, each leap perfectly timed. The wind is sharper here, cooler, carrying the scent of snow from higher peaks.

The music is at its peak, racing towards a final crescendo. You push with everything you have, sprinting the last stretch, until, in perfect sync with the music's final beat, you reach the summit. Standing there, chest heaving, heart pounding, you take in the breathtaking view, a sweeping panorama of mountains rolling into the distance, valleys shrouded in mist, and the sun casting long, golden beams across the peaks.

Hands on your hips, you breathe deeply, feeling the sheer vitality of the moment. You feel incredible, invincible. You've conquered the mountain, and it feels as if anything is possible. As you stand there, absorbing every detail of the stunning landscape, a deep, satisfying calm settles over you.

XXXIV

Dancing Through Seasons

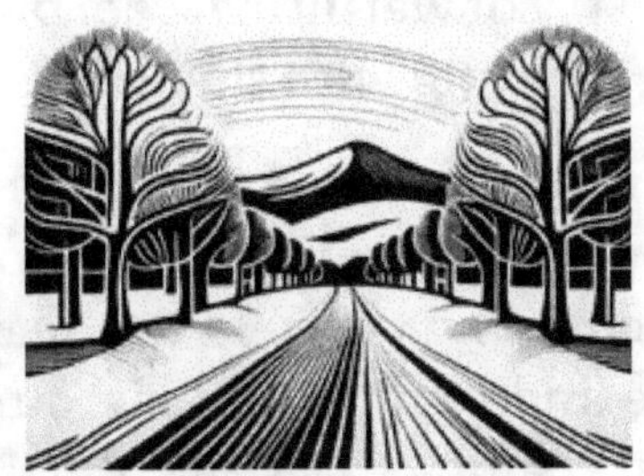

Allow yourself to drift into a scene where you are standing at the edge of a wide, open field in the gentle countryside. It's quiet here, and all around you, there's a sense of stillness, of simplicity. Before you stretches a wide swath of land, bordered by patches of woodlands, their trees a dark outline against the slowly lightening sky. Beyond, you catch the silhouette of a church spire from a distant village—a familiar shape reaching upward, marking the passage of centuries with its silent watch over the land.

As you look toward the horizon, the first light of dawn begins to spill softly across the landscape. The sky blushes in hues of lavender and gold, each cloud touched with a warm, gentle glow. Shadows lift from the ground, and every blade of grass, every budding leaf on the distant trees catches a glimmer of this early light, alive and fresh.

Then, something curious begins to happen. As you stand there, you notice that time itself seems to shift. The sun rises higher, faster than you'd expect, and the entire day unfolds before your eyes, flowing in a way that feels both natural and surreal. Morning gives way to the bright light of noon, casting long, warm shadows across the field. You feel the sun's heat and the richness of summer settle in, the air warm and filled with the scent of wildflowers and freshly cut hay.

But even this moment doesn't linger. Soon, the light begins to mellow, the sun sinking lower, casting a softer, amber glow. It's autumn now, and the trees on the distant edge of the field burst into vibrant colors; reds, oranges, and golds, transforming the landscape into a tapestry of warmth. A cool breeze stirs, and leaves drift across the field, swirling with the wind's gentle rhythm.

The scene shifts again, almost seamlessly. The colors fade to bare branches, the earth hardening as the air grows colder. A gentle snow begins to fall, covering the field in a blanket of quiet white, softening every edge and muffling every sound. You can feel the chill of winter here, its calm, reflective stillness.

And just as quickly, time shifts once more. The snow melts, revealing fresh, green shoots breaking through the earth. It's spring, and with it comes a sense of rebirth. The flowers bloom once again, the trees bud, and new life fills the field around you. Birds sing bright, early songs, and you feel the gentle touch of sunlight on your skin, warmer, bringing you back to where you began, at dawn.

As you take in these seasons passing in a breath, you realize you've stepped outside time as you know it. The days, weeks, and months blend seamlessly, all unfolding together in a cycle. You feel a profound sense of detachment from the ticking clock, from the pressure of hours and minutes. Here, there is only the flow of nature, a reminder that time itself is simply a concept, a way of measuring life, but not life itself.

With this awareness, you step outside your usual existence. You are no longer bound by time, by the need to rush or to keep up. Instead, you are a quiet observer of this eternal cycle, simply watching, experiencing, as each moment passes.

Take a deep breath, letting this perspective fill you. Know that whenever life feels rushed or pressured, you can return here in your mind's eye. Take this moment outside time and bring a piece of its calm, eternal presence back with you into your day.

XXXV

Garden of Gratitude

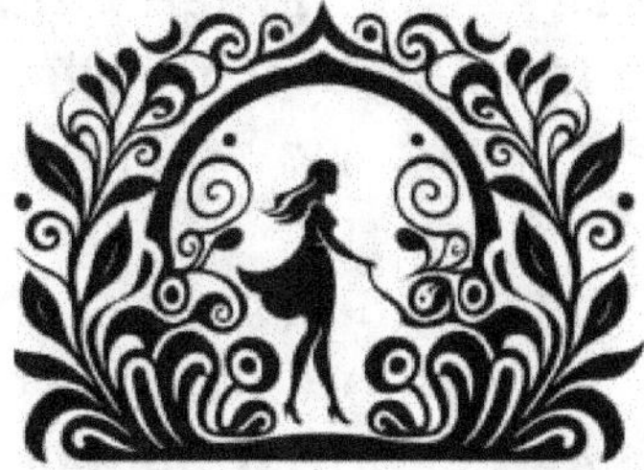

Close your eyes and imagine yourself standing at the edge of an ancient, beautiful forest, where sunlight filters gently through a canopy of towering trees. The air around you feels warm, a soft breeze drifting by and carrying with it the fresh scent of pine needles, earthy moss, and delicate wildflowers. In the distance, birds sing their morning songs, filling the air with sweet notes of calm and joy.

Before you, a moss-covered path stretches into the heart of the forest, lined with vibrant ferns and dappled with sunlight. This path seems to invite you forward, guiding you deeper into this enchanting landscape. As you step onto the soft ground, you can feel the earth beneath your feet, grounding you with each step. The colors around you seem to glow—the greens of leaves, the bright blossoms of wildflowers, each petal vivid and alive. And with every footfall, you feel yourself relaxing, leaving behind any worries as you are embraced by the peaceful energy of the forest.

After a while, you come across a small opening in the trees. Here, you discover a hidden space, a sacred haven known as the Gratitude Garden. It feels as if this garden has been created just for you, a place where every detail reflects a part of your heart. Stepping into this magical garden, you notice flowers blooming in radiant colors, lush greenery flourishing in every corner, and a gentle fountain at the center, its water trickling peacefully over smooth stones. The soft splash of water mingles with the bird songs, creating a soothing melody that fills the air.

You find a comfortable spot in this garden, perhaps a mossy stone bench or a soft patch of grass, and settle down, letting yourself relax fully. A wave of tranquility washes over you, as if the garden itself is wrapping you in a warm, loving embrace.

As you look around, you begin to realize that each flower here represents a moment of gratitude from your life; a cherished memory, a time when you felt loved, supported, or deeply joyful. Each bloom is a reminder of a gift life has given you, a gentle sign that you are never alone. Some flowers are small, some larger, each one unique, yet all grown from seeds of gratitude planted over time.

This inner garden, alive and thriving, is a reflection of the love and joy that fills your life, both past and present. With each positive thought, each grateful moment, this garden flourishes, growing more beautiful and abundant. In its blooms, you see the faces of loved ones, experiences of happiness, acts of kindness shared. This garden within you is always here, always blooming, ready to remind you of the strength and comfort found in gratitude.

Take a deep, cleansing breath, and feel the warmth of the sun shining down, the gentle caress of the breeze, and the comforting sense of your garden filling your heart. Let this feeling of gratitude radiate through you, bringing a smile to your face and a lightness to your being. Know that you can return to this peaceful place whenever you need to reconnect with your blessings and find peace.

When you're ready, bring your awareness back to your breath, noticing the gentle rise and fall of your chest. Feel the support of the ground beneath you, grounding you as you prepare to return to the present moment. Slowly, when you're ready, open your eyes, carrying with you a deep sense of gratitude and peace, ready to infuse your day with this beautiful feeling.

XXXVI

Echoes of the Sea

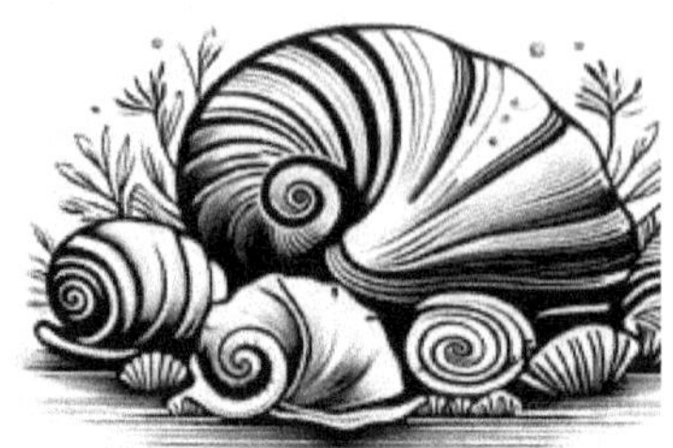

Picture yourself walking toward the beach as the sun begins its slow descent. The sand is warm beneath your feet, soft and inviting, molding gently to each step. A gentle breeze brushes past, carrying with it the faint scent of salt and sea, mingled with the warmth of the day's lingering heat. You're alone here, just you and the vast, open beach, the world quiet and calm around you.

Ahead, you see the ocean stretched out in front of you, waves rolling in a steady rhythm. Each one pulls and crashes gently, leaving a thin sheet of water that glides up the shore before receding, like a breath from the sea itself. You walk closer to the water's edge, and as you stand there, a larger wave reaches you, just brushing over your feet with coolness. The feeling is refreshing, grounding you in this serene, untouched place.

Looking out over the water, your eyes are drawn to the sun. It's a deep, vivid orange, hovering low over the horizon, an enormous ball casting golden hues across the sea's surface. The sunlight glints off the waves, scattering in sparks and glows as the sun dips lower, illuminating the world in shades of amber and rose.

You let your gaze wander down to the sand at your feet, stretching endlessly along the shore. It's fine and soft, a reminder of countless grains gathered over ages. As your eyes trace the beach stretching out in both directions, you marvel at the thought -

there must be thousands, perhaps millions, of grains right here, beneath you. Billions more stretching out along this beach alone, too many to count or imagine. It's impossible to grasp, a vast multitude, each grain a tiny piece of this immense landscape.

Kneeling down, you scoop a handful of sand, letting it sift slowly through your fingers. And as you look more closely, you notice that some grains aren't just sand, but minuscule seashells, delicate as jewels. Each is only a millimeter or two long, with intricate patterns and textures, some pale, others tinted with colors worn soft by the waves. Each one is beautiful, unique in its own way, like a world unto itself. And as you look at them, you find yourself wondering: How many of these tiny seashells are on this beach alone? Across all the beaches in the world? It's almost impossible to imagine—a beauty beyond comprehension.

You look up again, and the sun is now just touching the horizon, spreading wide and vast, a glowing orb that fills the sky. Its sheer size is humbling, as you recall that the sun could hold over a million Earths within it. And yet, it's just a single star among billions in the cosmos. You're surrounded by a universe so immense, so breathtaking in its scale and beauty, that words and thoughts seem to fall away.

In this moment, you feel a deep sense of awe and gratitude for being a part of something so vast, so extraordinary. Gently, you close your eyes, letting the stillness of the world around you settle into your mind. With each breath, you allow any thoughts to fade, letting go of anything beyond this moment. Here, in this calm, boundless place, you feel your mind begin to quiet.

Take a few breaths, feeling the immensity of the universe around you, holding you in its quiet embrace. As you listen to the waves and feel the sun's last warmth on your face, let your thoughts drift into the vastness, allowing yourself to be part of this peaceful, infinite beauty.

XXXVII

Frozen Grace

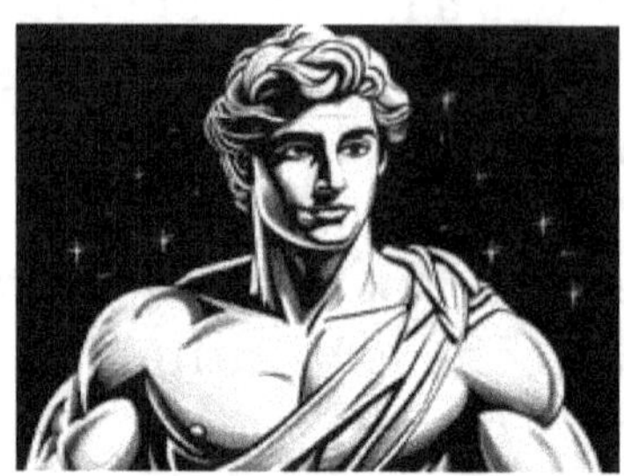

You drift into a dream where you find yourself in a spacious studio, lit by the gentle, honeyed light of morning. The studio's tall, arched windows stretch from floor to ceiling, allowing sunlight to stream in and spread across every surface, catching dust motes in the air and casting a warm, ethereal glow. The walls are painted a soft gray, heightening the quiet elegance of the space. Shelves line the studio's perimeter, displaying chisels, hammers, and an assortment of well-worn tools, each one awaiting the hand of a master.

Before you stands a massive, pristine slab of white marble; its surface a smooth, uninterrupted plane with faint swirls of pale blue and gray veining, like rivers beneath ice. You run your hand across its cool, solid expanse, feeling the promise it holds. Today, this stone will reveal something extraordinary.

Without a plan or sketch, you pick up your chisel, letting instinct guide you. You raise your hammer, and with the first sharp crack, you feel a surge of energy, as if the marble were whispering its secrets, ready to yield under your touch. Chip by chip, you carve with swift, practiced strokes, each movement effortless, guided by a force both familiar and mysterious. You lose all sense of time, the chisel in your hand becoming an extension of your will.

As you work, you remain unaware of the quiet footsteps

approaching, of people gathering around you, drawn by the rhythm of your hammer, by the beauty unfolding under your hands. Slowly, figures appear around the small platform you stand on, their eyes widening with fascination as they watch the marble transform.

Hours pass, though it feels like mere minutes. A figure begins to emerge: first the outline, then the strong, proud stance of a person, impossibly tall and perfect in form. You step back occasionally to observe, to refine, to breathe life into the shape. Legs, hips, the broad sweep of shoulders, each muscle appears defined, chiseled with such care that every contour and line feels alive, radiating a quiet strength.

Climbing a small stepladder, you reach the chest and sculpt the gentle curve of the ribs, the sculpted slope of the abdominal muscles, each detail embodying timeless beauty. Modesty requires a touch of tradition—a large leaf, artfully carved and placed. The audience is spellbound, their silence reverent as they witness the birth of something remarkable.

Finally, it's time for the face. With tender precision, you carve the profile: a strong jawline, a poised mouth, slightly parted as if to breathe, and eyes that carry strength and an undefinable softness. The beauty is captivating, a harmony of masculine power and an almost feminine grace. Your hands are steady, and you sense that this creation is now complete.

With one last, delicate scrape, you step down and gaze at your work. The audience stirs, murmurs breaking into gasps of awe, then applause. Hundreds of people are watching, their eyes reflecting admiration, some even awe-struck.

You step back, feeling a surge of pride and peace. In the stillness, a thought rises in your mind, a realization that every moment you spent here was a gift to your own spirit. This creation, born of your vision, skill, and dedication, is more than just stone shaped by hand. It's a testament to the boundless potential within you, proof that you hold the power to shape your life, your dreams, and your reality.

Take a deep breath and hold this feeling of accomplishment. Know that you are the sculptor of your own path, with the strength and creativity to create wonders, not just in stone, but in every choice you make.

XXXVIII

Sacred Steeple

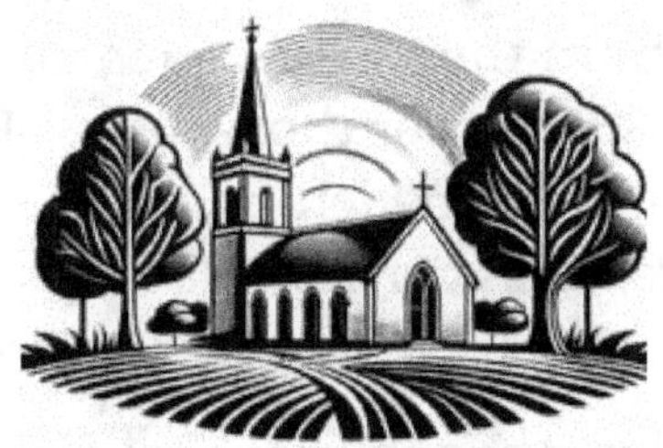

You find yourself standing at the entrance to an old village church, surrounded by an ancient graveyard where moss-covered stones tilt at odd angles, bearing the faint names of souls long gone. Many of the inscriptions are weathered beyond recognition, softened by time, though you can make out the occasional fragment: *Beloved… Departed…* Walking carefully through this quiet resting place, you feel the gentle weight of history around you, and even the air itself feels thick with memory.

As you approach the church's entrance, you notice the stone porch lined with faces carved into the walls, worn and softened by the elements but still faintly expressive—some solemn, others grimacing in a way that sends a chill down your spine. Their eyes, though hollowed by erosion, seem to follow you, like silent guardians of this sacred space.

Your hand reaches for the cold metal latch on the towering wooden door. It's heavy and solid, with the scars and grooves of centuries gone by. As you pull, the door creaks slowly, the sound resonating in the silence like a whispered invitation. Inside, the dim light filters through high arched windows, casting muted colors onto the stone floor. Dust particles float in the beams, creating a delicate haze, and the faint scent of wax and old wood fills the air.

The space is hushed and empty; you are the only soul here. This isn't a famous church, yet it is magnificent in its own quiet way. Tall stone columns line the aisle, standing like silent sentinels, and each one is carved with intricate designs. The nave stretches high above you, where beams adorned with small, carved figures seem to gaze down from their posts, each crafted with such care, as if meant to stand watch over those below. Rows of simple pews lead toward the altar, each bench polished smooth by countless hands over the years, each corner imbued with the reverence of those who came before.

As you walk slowly down the aisle, the faint echo of your footsteps seems to fall away, leaving only the silence. You reach the front of the church and settle into a pew, facing the altar, with its tall candles and faded cloths. The stained-glass windows tell stories you can't quite decipher, but the colors are striking, illuminated by the gentle morning light streaming through. Sitting here, it's impossible not to be moved by the sense of devotion embedded in this place.

In the stillness, you close your eyes and begin to meditate, finding it comes effortlessly. This space, steeped in hundreds of years of prayers and hopes, seems to invite you into a deeper state of reflection. Whether or not you share in the beliefs of those who built this church, you can sense that something profound resides here, a feeling as real as the stone beneath you. This building, from its foundation to its very spires, is woven with the energy of countless lives—people who came seeking solace, who poured out their joys, sorrows, and hopes within these walls.

It strikes you that, through time, others have sat right here, perhaps in desperation or gratitude, their quiet prayers adding to the invisible fabric that now seems to hold you gently, like an embrace. You feel connected to them, to each moment of whispered devotion and silent strength, the echoes of lives intersecting in this shared human experience.

With each breath, you find yourself more grounded, more attuned to the quiet wisdom of this place. A sense of calm wraps around you, a reminder that we are all, in some way, searching for connection, peace, and understanding. This sacred space could be a church, mosque, synagogue, or gurdwara—it doesn't matter what faith it represents, as they all carry the same essence of stillness and reflection. Here, in this timeless sanctuary, you feel your spirit joining the stream of countless others, united across time by a simple, shared humanity.

XXXIX

The Balance of Love

Close both eyes and take a deep breath. As you exhale, feel yourself stepping into a new scene. The warmth of the sun touches your skin, and you find yourself walking along a winding trail surrounded by rolling meadows. The air is crisp and fresh, carrying the delicate scent of wildflowers blooming in every color imaginable. Butterflies flit from bloom to bloom, their wings painted in vibrant hues, and the sound of birdsong fills the air, creating a melody of peace and joy.

Ahead, the path leads to a tranquil pond, its surface glimmering in the sunlight like liquid gold. The gentle rustling of the reeds at its edge is soothing, and the occasional ripple disturbs the otherwise perfect reflection of the sky above. You find a soft patch of grass near the water and settle down, stretching out as the beauty of the scene embraces you.

As you relax, you notice two ladybugs nearby. Their tiny, bright-red forms stand out against the green blades of grass. They move toward one another in a delicate, playful dance, their tiny legs brushing as they meet. You watch, captivated by their courtship, simple yet profound. One of them takes flight and lands gently on your hand, soon followed by the other. You smile, feeling their tiny presence on your skin.

You remember the old saying—that a ladybug is a sign of good luck, and two together might even mean a marriage within a year. But you shake the thought away with a chuckle. Marriage? Luck? You're far too busy for such things. Your days are filled with work, obligations, and always being there for others. Yet, as the ladybugs take flight again, you can't help but feel a small tug in your heart, as though they've left a subtle message behind.

Your gaze shifts to the pond, where two elegant swans glide across the water. Their movements are effortless, a dance in perfect synchrony. They bow their heads toward one another, and for a fleeting moment, their necks form the unmistakable shape of a heart. They seem entirely unaware of your presence, lost in their shared world.

You think of someone in your life; a person who's shown interest, kindness, perhaps even love. You've kept them at arm's length, telling yourself there's no time for such nonsense. But watching the swans, their bond so palpable, you can't deny the beauty of their connection.

As you reflect, two playful dogs come bounding along the path. Their tails wag with enthusiasm as they frolic together, nipping and tumbling in joyous abandon. They notice you sitting on the grass and run toward you, their eyes shining with affection.

You reach out to pet them, and they eagerly press their warm bodies against you, soaking up your touch. Their happiness is infectious, and for a moment, you're simply present, sharing in their joy. But as they nuzzle closer, something shifts. Their attention feels different—not just playful, but deliberate. They seem to be offering you something more, something you can't quite name.

Eventually, they trot off together, their tails swaying in harmony. You watch them go, a pang of something unspoken lingering in your chest. Have you been so focused on giving to others; your time, your care, your love—that you've forgotten how to receive it?

A gentle breeze stirs the air around you, and you close your eyes, hearing its quiet whisper. Giving and receiving are like the breath: both are essential, and both must flow in balance. Just as the world around you thrives in harmony, so too does love.

Perhaps it's time to open your heart; to let love not only flow outward but also inward. As you take a deep breath, imagine yourself inhaling love and acceptance from the world around you, and as you exhale, let it flow back out, stronger and brighter.

XL

Flow & Stillness

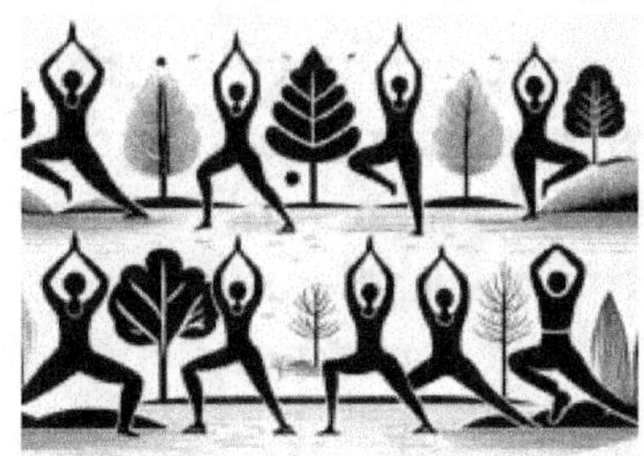

You can see yourself entering a light-filled yoga hall, polished wooden floors gleaming beneath your feet, walls painted in calm earth tones that seem to breathe with warmth. The air carries a subtle hint of incense, mixed with the freshness of the morning, and soft instrumental music plays faintly in the background. The sunlight filters through the large, arched windows, casting delicate patterns on the floor and creating a peaceful atmosphere where shadows dance along with the light. You feel a sense of calm envelop you as you settle onto your mat, surrounded by others who seem equally eager to dive into practice.

The teacher, a graceful young woman with an ease and fluidity in her movements, begins to guide the class. She demonstrates the poses with precision, her body flowing effortlessly from one posture to the next. Around you, other practitioners mirror her with practiced grace, moving in a perfect rhythm, seemingly without strain. Their bodies bend with agility, stretching long and low into postures you remember being able to hold more easily in years past.

You follow along, doing your best, but you find yourself adjusting the poses here and there, choosing gentler variations. You pause, noticing the contrast between yourself and the others who appear so confident in their strength and flexibility. There's a subtle, fleeting feeling of being out of sync, a whisper of self-consciousness that arises as you consider how you might look to others in the room. Are they noticing? Judging? A pang of discomfort settles briefly in your chest, but you push it away and focus on your breath.

Yet, as you glance around, you realize there is no critical gaze upon you. The teacher, radiating kindness, moves close and offers you an encouraging nod, her eyes soft and reassuring. She doesn't push or correct but offers subtle adjustments to help you settle into your own version of each pose. In those quiet moments, you sense an understanding between you both; an unspoken acknowledgment that this practice is unique for everyone.

As the class draws to a close, you lie back for savasana, closing your eyes and letting the weight of your body sink deeply into the mat. Here, in this final relaxation, you feel at home, as if you've found your place. The rise and fall of your breath fills your awareness, and a wave of relaxation washes over you, deeper than any asana, enveloping you in a stillness that feels like pure presence. This is where you truly connect, where you find the essence of yoga. Your body, mind, and breath come together, and the judgments and comparisons of before seem to fade, leaving only peace.

After class, you hear two other participants chatting softly as they roll up their mats, expressing surprise at the relaxation at the end. "I don't get why we lie there for so long," one says, laughing lightly. "I'd rather just keep moving."

A quiet realization settles over you, deepening as you listen. Flexibility and physical movement are just one part of yoga's vast landscape. Yoga isn't a race or competition; it's a space for self-awareness, a journey to listen to your body and your inner voice. You reflect on how the deeper, quieter aspects of yoga—like savasana—are where you truly excel. You begin to see the class through new eyes, realizing that the stillness, the mindfulness, is as valuable as any physical prowess.

Yoga, you realize, is not about being "good" or reaching for perfection. It's not a sport where some succeed and others fail. There is no goal other than being here in this moment, connecting inward. And it dawns on you that, asana is just one small part of the whole; a gateway to something much more profound. As you gather your things, you leave with a new sense of calm and contentment, carrying the quiet wisdom of yoga within you, knowing you've touched something much deeper than movement alone.

XLI

Charon

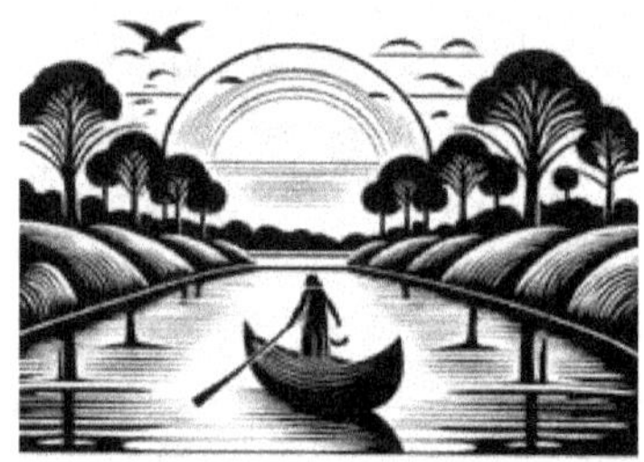

Imagine yourself standing on a desolate, mist-shrouded riverbank, where the air feels thick, almost heavy, and a quiet chill wraps around you. The River Styx stretches out before you, a wide, slow-moving expanse of dark water, its surface glistening with faint ripples. Wisps of mist curl and dance above the river, swirling as though moved by unseen spirits. It is an otherworldly silence, thick and profound, and you sense that this is no ordinary river—it is a boundary, a place of passage between realms.

Before you, an ancient ferry creaks against the shoreline, tethered by nothing more than a fraying rope. Standing in the shadows is Charon, the ferryman, his form cloaked in a worn, dark robe that obscures his face. With a steady hand, he gestures for you to step aboard, his silent presence both formidable and calm. You feel compelled to accept his invitation, knowing that this journey is part of your destiny.

You step onto the ferry, and it rocks gently underfoot, echoing with the soft groan of wood meeting water. Charon pushes off from the shore, and as he does, you settle into the boat, feeling the weight of the river's gravity pull you deeper into the mist. The ferry drifts forward, and all around you is quiet, a silence so vast it absorbs even the smallest sound, as if the river itself is alive, listening, and holding your presence within its depths.

As the ferry glides over the dark water, you feel the mist surrounding you, cool and damp, brushing against your skin like faint memories. The river feels almost timeless, as if it has existed since the dawn of creation. You realize that this river, the Styx, represents the divide between life and what lies beyond. It is the boundary between the familiar world of the living and the mysteries of what comes after, a sacred passage that countless souls have crossed before you.

You find yourself gazing deeply into the water, where fleeting glimpses of faces seem to appear, only to dissolve into the depths again—echoes of the lives that have passed through this realm. This is not a place of fear but a space of quiet reflection, and you find yourself surrendering to the slowness of this crossing, allowing the river to carry you forward.

Charon stands at the helm, guiding the boat with practiced hands, his face obscured yet somehow familiar, as though he is both stranger and guardian. You feel safe in his silent presence, as though he understands the significance of this journey without words. You begin to sense that this crossing is not just about an end but about the continuity of all that has come before and all that will follow.

The mist begins to thin, revealing a distant shore, cloaked in shadow but softened by a faint, gentle light. As you approach, you sense a deep stillness within yourself, a quiet acceptance of all that has been and all that must be released. You are reminded of the fleeting nature of life, of how each breath, each heartbeat, has been a gift, precious and ephemeral.

Now, as the ferry reaches the other shore, you look back at the river, at the swirling mist that conceals so many memories, moments, and lives. You understand that, like the river's currents, your journey has been a series of waves and ripples, ever-shifting but always moving forward. You realize that this journey is not an end but a transformation, a moment of release, of surrender to the natural cycle.

Charon turns to you, and though he says nothing, his presence imparts a feeling of reverence for all you have lived and all that you leave behind. With a final nod, you step from the ferry, feeling a lightness, a sense of peace and completion. You are ready to let go, to move forward into whatever lies beyond, knowing that your life, like every life, was a beautiful, transient ripple in the great river of existence.

And as you turn, you carry with you a quiet, profound understanding that the journey of life is sacred, each moment an echo, a memory, etched into the river's timeless flow. You return to the present moment, opening your eyes with a sense of peace, gratitude, and acceptance of all that is.

XLII

Silver Screen

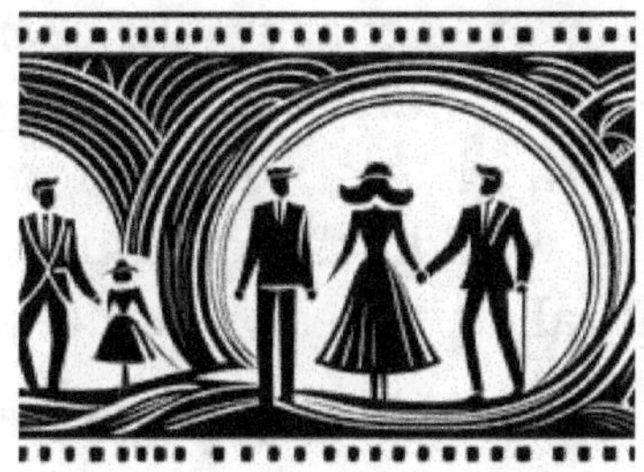

You find yourself on a quiet evening, flipping through the channels or scrolling through a streaming service, only to realize there's nothing new that truly grabs your interest. Eventually, almost resignedly, you settle on an old black-and-white movie. It's a film you might never have chosen on your own, perhaps an old noir or a romance with the slight tint of nostalgia. The actors, with their carefully groomed hair and old-school mannerisms, seem vaguely familiar; their names ring faint bells, remnants of a time when they were once household names, now all but forgotten.

As the film begins, you find yourself adjusting to the slower pacing, the grainy monochrome, and the occasional flicker of the frame—a product of another era. For the first few minutes, you watch with mild detachment, a part of you tempted to switch it off, but something holds you back. Then, subtly, you find yourself being drawn into the story, caught off guard by the simplicity and charm of a plot that unravels with a patience you don't often see in modern films. It's nothing extraordinary, no world-saving superhero, no apocalyptic stakes—just a story of everyday people, navigating relatable challenges and emotions. Before you know it, the simplicity has pulled you in, and you're engrossed.

The characters move and speak with a kind of grace that feels almost foreign now, a relic from a time when men were men and women were women. The male characters are sturdy and steady, their expressions a mixture of resolve and subtle vulnerability, while the female characters carry themselves with a sort of unspoken elegance. Their language, too, belongs to a different time. You might cringe slightly at phrases that feel awkward by today's standards, words that might seem outdated or even a bit uncomfortable now, but you let it pass. These actors are playing roles written in an era with different values, different assumptions about the world. It's a curious snapshot of history, a glimpse into the cultural attitudes of the past.

And then, the film takes an unexpected turn—a suspenseful moment, perhaps, or a bit of action. It's the kind of scene that, in a modern movie, would come with a full orchestra of sound effects, digital explosions, and dizzying camera angles. But here, the "special effects" are charmingly humble, a touch theatrical, almost naïve. An explosion might be represented by little more than a burst of smoke, a car chase by a few quick cuts and shaky close-ups. And yet, the anticipation is there. There's something deeply satisfying about the build-up, the way the characters' tension mounts, each scene designed to draw you in rather than overwhelm you. The sparing use of these moments somehow makes them more impactful, a far cry from the relentless action we're used to today. You're reminded that sometimes, the imagination fills in the blanks far better than high-tech wizardry.

As the credits roll, you're left with a surprising sense of satisfaction. Watching the movie felt like slipping into a time capsule, briefly living in an era vastly different from our own, and you're glad for the experience. In some ways, it's refreshing —a reprieve from the sensory overload of modern blockbusters, a reminder that there's more than one way to tell a story. But you're also aware that, while this journey into the past was enjoyable, you wouldn't want it to be your only experience. You appreciate the advancements in film that bring extraordinary worlds to life with such vivid detail. Both the old and the new have their place; it's not a matter of better or worse, but a balance.

In this way, people are like that, too. Speak to someone much older or much younger than yourself, and it can feel almost as though you're speaking to someone from another time—a different generation with different perspectives and experiences. The wisdom and groundedness of the older generation offer a steadying anchor, a sense of continuity and history. Meanwhile, the young bring passion, energy, and a refreshing optimism, often seeing the world with fresh eyes and boundless enthusiasm. Each group has its place, each bringing something valuable to the table. The older generation, like those classic films, offer perspective and depth, while the young, like modern movies, keep life dynamic and evolving.

Just as you wouldn't want to limit yourself to only watching old movies or exclusively new ones, life feels richer with both the wisdom of experience and the spark of new possibilities. Together, they make for a more complete, fulfilling experience—a balance that feeds your passion for life.

Within the Earth

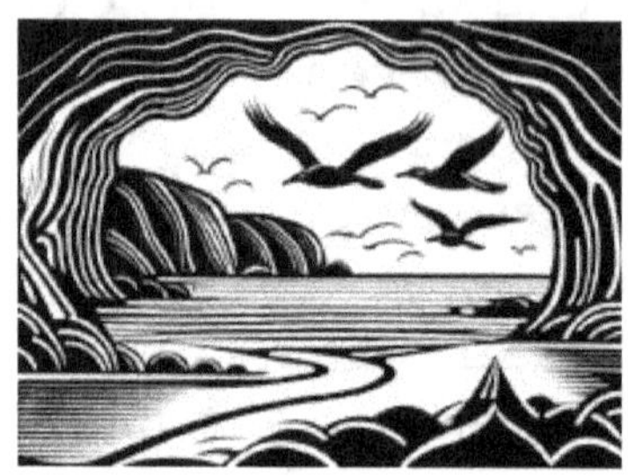

Close your eyes and allow yourself to sink into a state of relaxation, letting your breath move slowly and deeply. Picture yourself standing alone on a remote, sandy beach, a hidden cove where the world feels untouched and calm. The soft golden sand is warm underfoot, and the rhythmic sound of gentle waves laps against the shore. The air carries a hint of salt, mingling with the scent of sun-warmed rock. You take in a deep breath, savoring the clean ocean breeze, and feel the sun's gentle warmth on your skin, its rays casting a soft golden glow on the world around you.

You settle onto the sand, feeling the peace of solitude and the vastness of the ocean stretching out before you. Time seems to slow as you gaze out, letting each wave rise and fall like the steady rhythm of your breath. But as the waves come and go, you suddenly realize that the tide has crept in without your noticing, filling the cove and blocking your way back along the beach. The cliffs behind you rise steeply, their craggy faces slick with salt and seaweed, unscalable without a proper path.

Noticing a dry patch at the back of the cove, you decide to wait there until the tide retreats. But as you turn to settle against the rock face, a seabird, a sleek, silvery gull, calls loudly from above, circling and swooping close. The bird's calls become more persistent, almost urgent, as it flits down toward the far end of the cove. You wonder if it has a nest nearby, but there's no nest between you and the water. The gull keeps darting toward a shadowy area at the base of the cliff, catching your attention with its unrelenting cries.

Curious, you follow the bird's path to where it seems to disappear into the cliff itself. You step closer and notice a fissure in the rock, barely wide enough for you to squeeze through. You feel a strange pull to explore, a curiosity sparked by the gull's insistence, so you carefully slip inside. The narrow crack opens up unexpectedly, revealing a space within; a small path of smooth stones leading upward, beckoning you deeper into the cliff.

To your surprise, the cave has a faint, natural glow. The rocks emit a soft, ethereal light, bathing the walls in hues of pale green and silvery blue, illuminating your way without need of any torch. You begin to climb, taking in the cave's beauty; the gentle glow reflects off gleaming stalactites hanging like crystal daggers from the ceiling, dripping water that echoes softly in the cavern. Beneath you, stalagmites rise like silent guardians, some of them forming columns where they've met their partners above. The air is cool and carries a faint, earthy scent, grounding and refreshing, as if the cave itself breathes along with you.

The path twists and narrows in some places, but it always seems to lead upward. Though you're deep within the cliff, a sense of safety and calmness settles over you, and any fears or doubts fade away as you climb. After several minutes, you notice a soft light spilling through an opening ahead. The gull appears once more, perched by a gap in the rock, watching as you approach. As you reach the opening, the gull flutters up and out, flying into the sky. You follow, emerging into the sunlight at the very top of the cliff.

Stepping into the open air, you're greeted by a panoramic view of the ocean, its vast expanse glistening in the sunlight far below. The gull is nowhere to be seen. You glance down at the grassy cliff edge, searching for the cave entrance you came from, but it's vanished; only smooth grass remains. For a moment, you're struck by a feeling of wonder, as if the cave, the path, and the gentle glow were part of a strange dream.

In this quiet moment, a gentle thought arises, an insight like the soft glow that led you upward: perhaps safety and guidance can come in unexpected forms, from places within ourselves we don't always recognize. The path to safety, to clarity, sometimes appears only when we step forward into the unknown, trusting something beyond sight or reason. Standing alone on the clifftop, you breathe in deeply, feeling the warmth of gratitude and the mystery of life's hidden pathways. And with that sense of wonder and calm, you carry this peace back with you, allowing the image to slowly dissolve as you return to the present moment.

XLIV

Savasana II

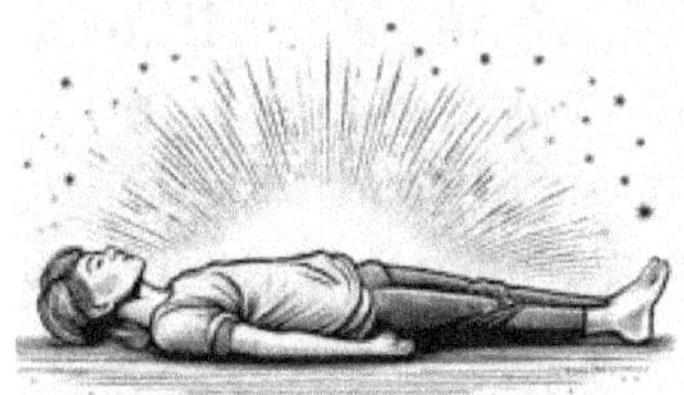

Lie down comfortably on your mat, letting your entire body settle. Stretch out your legs and let your feet relax open to the sides. Rest your arms gently at your sides, with your palms facing upward, ready to receive. Adjust yourself until you feel a sense of ease and balance.

Close your eyes and take a long, slow breath in…and as you exhale, let go of any lingering tension. Feel yourself gradually melting into the support of the mat. Each breath brings a deeper sense of heaviness, of surrender to the present moment. Allow your body to feel fully supported, embraced by the earth beneath you, as if you could let every muscle rest and release.

Now, begin to imagine a gentle, golden light hovering just above your feet. This light is warm, calm, and comforting, radiating a soft glow. With your next breath, visualize this golden light entering your body through the soles of your feet, bringing a sense of warmth and relaxation. Let the light flow through your toes, gently wrapping around each one, and feel a deep sense of comfort spreading from your toes into your entire foot. With each breath, this light invites calmness, releasing any tension.

The golden light now begins to flow up to your ankles, wrapping them in warmth and ease. Sense your ankles softening, any tightness dissolving, as you exhale gently. The light continues to rise, flowing up into your calves, where it fills each muscle, melting away any remaining tension. Each exhale encourages a deeper sense of relaxation, allowing your legs to feel heavy, comfortable, and perfectly at rest.

Now, feel this gentle warmth reaching your knees and gradually moving up to your thighs. The golden light fills every muscle here, soothing and releasing. Any tightness you may be holding slowly fades away, and your legs feel completely relaxed, sinking heavily into the mat. Your breath is natural, steady, and light, each one allowing you to let go a little more.

The light flows upward, reaching your hips, moving through your pelvis and lower back. Feel the warmth and relaxation spread through this entire area, releasing any stress or tension held here. Each breath brings an even greater sense of ease, allowing your body to soften further, melting into the mat as this calming golden light fills your lower body.

Now, sense the light moving up into your abdomen, gently warming and soothing every part of you from the inside out. Your belly softens, and with it, a feeling of deep peace spreads through your entire torso. Imagine each breath helping this light to expand, to radiate through every cell, gently encouraging a state of ease and quiet.

As the light rises to your chest, feel it filling your heart with warmth and calm. Your breath slows, and each inhalation feels light, effortless. The golden light soothes your chest, bringing a comforting sense of relaxation, as though every heartbeat is bathed in warmth. Allow yourself to fully receive this peace, to let it settle deeply within.

The golden light now moves up to your shoulders, melting away any burdens you may be carrying. Imagine this light flowing down each arm, filling your upper arms, softening your elbows, and then moving down to your forearms, wrists, and finally to the very tips of your fingers. Let your hands rest in this gentle warmth, allowing any last bits of tension to simply slip away.

Feel the light return to your shoulders, then gently rise up through your neck, easing away any tightness, allowing your throat to soften. The warmth continues upward, flowing along your jaw, relaxing the muscles there, then up into your cheeks, soothing your eyes, and finally settling at the very top of your head.

Your entire body is now bathed in golden light, a gentle warmth filling every part of you. There's a deep, calm energy moving through you, and you feel a profound sense of ease, as though every part of you is at rest, perfectly at peace.

Allow yourself to linger here, breathing gently, held by this light, supported by the earth beneath you. There's nowhere else you need to be, nothing you need to do. Simply rest in this light, letting it cradle you, nurturing every part of you with calm and warmth.

When you're ready, begin to bring your awareness back, slowly, gently. Notice the sensation of your body on the mat, the air around you, the rhythm of your breath. You may start to wiggle your fingers and toes, and when you feel ready, take a deep breath and return to the room, carrying this golden warmth with you.

XLV

The Sage

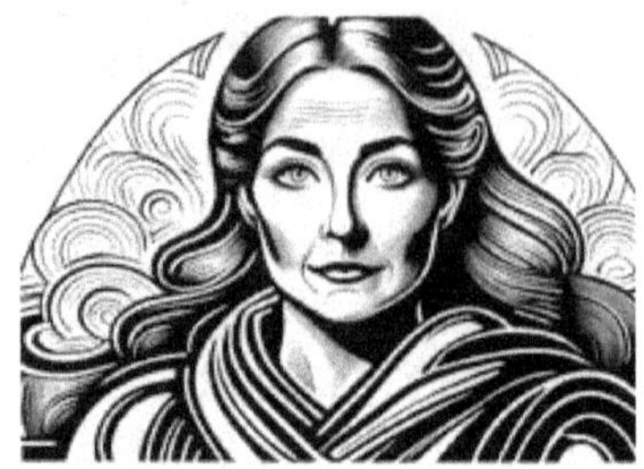

Take a deep breath and gently close your eyes. Picture yourself in the heart of towering mountains, surrounded by the vastness of their ridges and peaks stretching toward the sky.The air here is so clear, it feels like a gift with every inhale, crisp and pure, filling your lungs with a refreshing chill. You are on a solitary path, winding through rocks and patches of scree, and with each step, you feel the rugged terrain beneath your feet, grounding you deeply in this moment, in this place.

Your journey is long, winding upwards along narrow trails that twist around steep slopes, leading ever closer to the realm of the clouds. The path is uneven, sometimes giving way to wild patches of snowfields where your steps leave soft imprints. The silence of the mountains surrounds you, punctuated only by the occasional call of distant birds or the soft crunch of your footsteps in the snow. Each step brings you closer, through the solitude of this ancient landscape, toward something unknown yet deeply familiar.

As you make your way up a final ridge, you catch sight of a small, weathered hut nestled into the side of the mountain. The hut is humble and worn, its roof barely visible beneath layers of draped prayer flags, tattered by the wind, yet vibrant in their faded colors. The flags ripple gently, sending whispers through the air. Wind chimes dangle near the doorway, each gust causing them to sing soft, eerie notes that seem to dance on the breeze, as if welcoming you to this hidden refuge.

You approach the hut, and as you near the threshold, the old wooden door swings open with a gentle creak, as if expecting you. You step inside and are immediately enveloped in a world of shadow and quiet. The air is thick with the scent of incense, curling in delicate trails that drift around the room, cloaking it in a mysterious haze. In the center of the room, sitting cross-legged on a simple mat, is a figure wrapped in dark robes. Their hood is pulled low, obscuring their face entirely, shrouding them in shadow.

For a moment, you stand there in silence, captivated by this figure —this sage whom you have traveled so far to meet. Without a word, they gesture for you to sit, a gentle sweep of the hand inviting you to join them. You move toward the mat in front of them and settle down, feeling the coldness of the stone floor beneath you.

In front of the sage is a small pot of green tea. With a fluid, practiced motion, they pour two cups, the tea steaming gently in the cool air. They hand you one of the cups, and you take it, feeling the warmth of it radiate through your fingers. You sip, and the tea's warmth spreads through you, both soothing and invigorating, a quiet moment of refreshment after your long journey. You nod gratefully and whisper a soft, "Thank you."

You sit together in silence, the kind of silence that feels thick, charged with meaning. You came here seeking answers, wisdom, perhaps a sign to guide you on your path. You clear your throat, preparing to speak, to ask the questions you've held inside. But before a single word can escape, the sage lifts a hand, a gesture to hold back your questions, to silence the words that form on your lips.

Then, slowly, almost ceremonially, the sage raises both hands to their hood. They pull it back, and as the shadow falls away, you see their face. You catch your breath, stunned, for you are staring back at yourself.

The realization settles over you like a gentle dawn. You understand, in that moment, that the answers you sought were never outside of you. The wisdom, the guidance, the clarity—they have always been within. You are both the seeker and the sage. You hold the questions, and you hold the answers.

In this quiet space, you feel a sense of peace, a deep knowing that you already possess what you need to guide your journey forward. The sage before you is merely a reflection, a reminder that your inner teacher has always been present, waiting for you to recognize it.

You take one last sip of the tea, savoring its warmth, its simplicity, before gently setting the cup down. The figure before you nods, as if acknowledging this newfound understanding. In the silence that follows, you feel a profound connection to yourself, to this wisdom that resides within.

For a few moments, you sit in stillness, letting the knowledge sink into the very depths of your being.

XLVI

The Dance of Colors

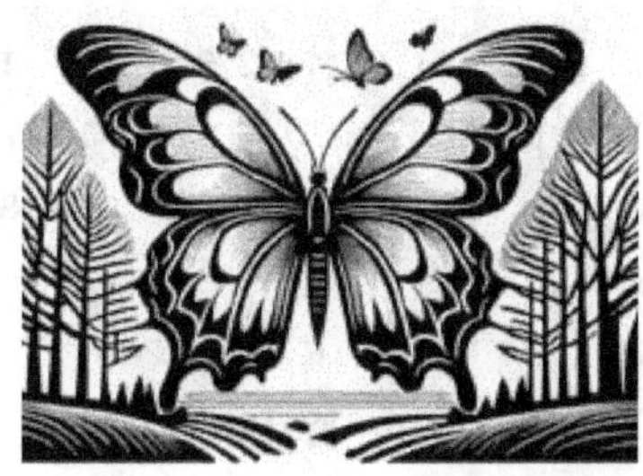

Visualize yourself in a gray, misty town where the streets are damp and quiet. Buildings of faded brick and worn paint line narrow roads, their colors muted by the overcast sky. The air is still, a bit chilly, carrying the faint hum of distant traffic, as if life here has settled into a slow, steady rhythm. You walk through a small town park, where patches of patchy grass and bare-limbed trees are scattered across a stretch of concrete paths and benches. A pair of pigeons peck listlessly near a puddle, adding to the somber mood of the place.

As you move deeper into the park, you spot a small butterfly; a modest creature with plain, brown wings, so subtle it almost blends into the background. Its fluttering catches your eye, and you decide to follow it, feeling a sudden curiosity as it leads you along a winding path lined with sparse bushes. The butterfly pauses on a leaf, fluttering in a delicate dance as if acknowledging your presence before it flits off again. Just as it disappears from view, another butterfly appears, this one a striking shade of blue, delicate and shimmering with a hint of iridescence. It hovers nearby, circling and weaving gracefully in the air.

This blue butterfly leads you further, gliding ahead with a soft elegance. Soon, you come upon an orange butterfly with intricate patterns on its wings, vibrant as a painted canvas. It looks as though nature herself took extra care to adorn this one with splashes of earthy orange and deep black lines. The orange butterfly flutters around the blue, and they spin together in a beautiful spiral before the blue one darts up high, vanishing into the sky. You follow the orange butterfly, which drifts toward the outskirts of town, guiding you as if on a gentle breeze.

As you leave the park and enter the edge of the countryside, the air feels lighter, and you notice a break in the clouds. Sunlight starts to filter through, warming the landscape and casting a golden glow on the fields and hedgerows around you. You can see a winding path bordered by wildflowers, their vibrant colors a delightful contrast to the gray town behind you. The scent of fresh earth and blossoming flowers fills the air, and a feeling of peace settles over you.

Just ahead, another butterfly appears, its wings a rich tapestry of deep reds and velvety blacks with a few white spots that catch the sunlight. This new butterfly dances around the orange one, their movements graceful as if they're performing a duet. They seem almost to be speaking, exchanging a message carried on the wind. Then, as if bidding farewell, the orange butterfly floats high, disappearing into the sky, leaving you with the red and black beauty to guide your way.

You follow this butterfly down a trail that leads into an open meadow. The sky is now bright, and the sun bathes the landscape in warm light. Grasses sway gently in the breeze, dotted with wildflowers in shades of yellow, purple, and white. Birds chirp from nearby trees, and the land feels alive, humming with the energy of nature. The butterfly flits through the meadow, and in its company, you feel a growing sense of connection to the beauty around you.

Ahead, a new butterfly appears; an exquisite creature with large, pale yellow wings bordered with inky black lines and a hint of deep blue near its body. Its wings are broad and regal, seeming almost to command the air as it glides effortlessly beside the red butterfly. They twirl and circle each other, as if sharing a silent, timeless language known only to them. After a moment, the red butterfly ascends, disappearing into the light-dappled sky, leaving you to continue following the elegant yellow butterfly.

Your journey leads you to a peaceful pond nestled within a small grove of trees. Sunlight filters through the canopy of silver birch and Scots pine, casting dappled shadows on the water's surface. Bullrushes stand tall along the banks, and dragonflies zip around, their iridescent wings flashing in the sunlight. The pond's surface is glassy, reflecting the sky above and the branches that arch protectively overhead. The yellow butterfly lands softly on a moss-covered log beside the water, as if inviting you to rest.

You settle down on the log, gazing at the pond, its surface calm and undisturbed. The butterfly remains beside you, a gentle companion on this journey. Closing your eyes, you allow the sounds of nature to fill your mind; the soft rustle of leaves, the gentle splash of a fish breaking the surface, the buzzing of dragonflies. In this moment, you sense a quiet message: Life, like the butterflies, leads you forward in gentle stages. Each step, each encounter, has its own beauty, guiding you from the gray into the light. You feel a deep calm, a renewed appreciation for the small wonders that reveal themselves when you follow life's quiet, subtle invitations.

XLVII

Tale of Two Villages

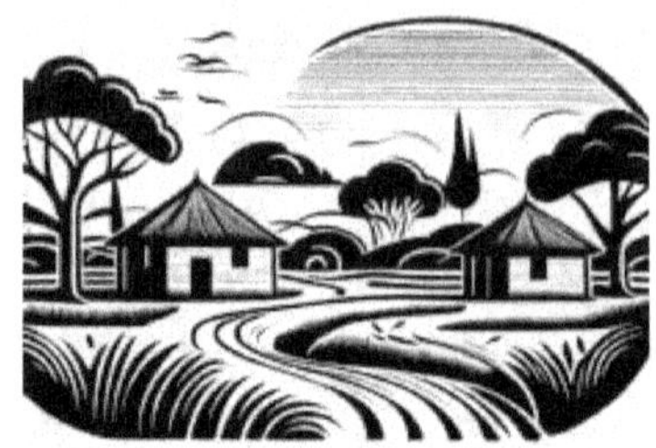

Close your eyes and start to relax into your breath. Let each inhale fill you with calm, and each exhale release any tension in your body. Picture yourself setting off on a journey, backpack on, walking through a foreign countryside far from home. The sun is low in the sky, casting a warm, golden glow over the landscape as you travel, your feet pressing into the dry, dusty earth with each step. You're tired, hungry, and thirsty. Your journey has been long, and the comforts of home feel distant.

As you walk, you begin to see the faint outline of a village on the horizon; a scattering of small, makeshift houses and humble shacks surrounded by fields and open land. Drawing closer, you notice the worn, patched materials and the simple designs, a place without frills or luxuries, yet full of character and resilience. An underfed dog raises its head, barking faintly to announce your arrival. The few villagers nearby look up, their faces curious but cautious, unaccustomed to visitors. The children are the first to break the silence. A small group gathers at a distance, peeking at you with wide eyes, their intrigue overcoming their shyness. They inch closer and, one by one, start to smile, then giggle among themselves, as if you're the most fascinating sight they've seen in days.

You smile back, nodding gently to them, and even though you don't speak their language, the air fills with a sense of connection.

Children tug at your shirt, some reaching for your hand, pulling you closer. You feel their tiny hands in yours and remember the sweets in your pocket; barely enough, but you offer one to each of them. Their joy is overwhelming, eyes sparkling with excitement at this small gesture. Laughter fills the air, lifting your spirit as you watch them savor the sweets as if they were the finest treats in the world.

Suddenly, a ball rolls towards your feet, and the children beckon you to join their game. You want to play along, to share in their lightness, but exhaustion holds you back. Just then, a man approaches, kindly waving the children away and gesturing for you to follow him. You walk slowly behind, feeling a wave of relief, and he leads you into one of the modest homes. Inside, a family sits in a circle, and they make room for you in the honored spot; a humble gesture of respect. A woman serves you sweet tea, pouring it into a cup that she refills almost as soon as you finish it. You feel the warmth of the tea reviving you, filling the empty ache in your belly.

After a few moments, they bring you a simple yet nourishing meal; food that tastes beyond anything you've had before, each bite warming your core and sating the hunger that had been gnawing at you. You eat slowly, realizing someone here may have given up their own portion for you. When you decline a second helping, a quiet sadness falls over the room. Sensing this, you nod and accept more, honoring their hospitality. Eventually, you sink back, letting your eyes close, intending just to rest - but sleep overtakes you, wrapped in the warm energy of their home.

You awake to gentle, watchful faces. As you sit up, you realize your backpack has been left untouched by your side. Your mind flashes to your passport and money, and you feel a pang of guilt for even questioning its safety. The family watches you with understanding, a silent reassurance that you were safe here. You smile and prepare to leave, offering a gesture of thanks with money from your wallet. But they gently wave it away, shaking their heads with firm dignity. To press the matter would be disrespectful. Overwhelmed by their kindness, you offer a bow of gratitude, your heart full yet heavy as you walk away.

The sun is dipping lower, and your thoughts turn to a walk you took once back home, remembering how you were tired and thirsty as you passed a village of opulent homes. You see the image clearly in your mind, the lush gardens, the manicured lawns, the shining cars. As you passed by, you noticed the cautious stares and averted eyes. Needing water, you approached a man hosing down his pristine car. Politely, you asked for a bit of water to refill your bottle. He frowned and dismissed you with a curt "No," turning his back without a second thought.

You shake your head, remembering the contrast, the people who had so much yet shared so little. In this moment, you're left wondering why those with so little can give so freely, while those with so much can be reluctant to share. A feeling of quiet wisdom settles over you. True wealth, you realize, is not found in what we possess, but in what we're willing to share.

As you let these thoughts settle, take a deep breath in, feeling gratitude for the kindness of strangers, the richness of simple moments, and the abundance that exists when hearts are open. Let that sense of deep gratitude fill your being as you breathe out, grounding you in the beauty of humility and generosity.

XLVIII

Silent Observer

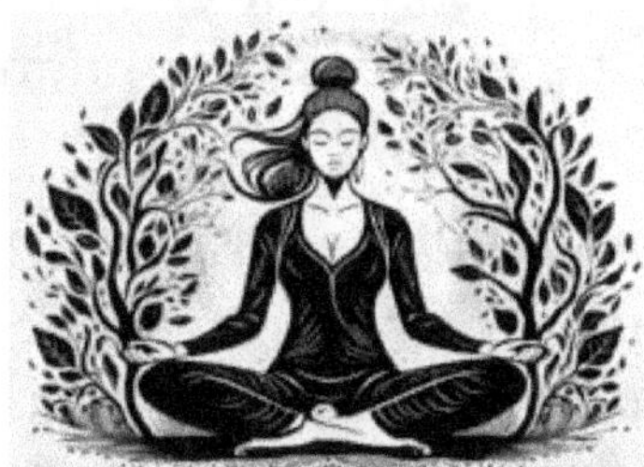

Breathe deeply as you notice your eyelids grow heavy and let your body relax completely. Feel the gentle weight of gravity grounding you to the earth. Take a deep breath in through your nose, and as you exhale, release any tension in your shoulders, your jaw, and your mind. Allow yourself to step into a vivid mental scene: a place where calm and clarity surround you completely.

It's a fine day, one you've been anticipating for several mornings. The rain and wind of the past few days have kept you indoors, but today, the sun is shining, and the air feels fresh and welcoming. As has become your habit, you prepare for your outdoor meditation, a ritual you've come to treasure.

You find yourself walking to a special place, a quiet and overgrown section of the local cemetery. Far from eerie, this place is alive with the sounds of birdsong and the subtle rustle of leaves. It is a space that exudes warmth and a quiet sense of welcome, as though the souls resting here are glad to have their solitude shared peacefully.

As you make your way through your neighborhood, you pull out your phone and briefly glance at your social media. There it is: a sharp, biting comment under something you posted. The words are intentionally unkind, meant to provoke. For a moment, you feel the pull to respond, to defend yourself, to argue. But as you stand there, phone in hand, you remember other such exchanges; how they escalated, how they drained your energy and left you unsettled.

Instead, you close the app and take a deep breath. You've decided that today, you will not let someone else's negativity invade your peace. With a final swipe, you tuck your phone away and continue walking.

The day is glorious. Sunlight streams through the trees, and a soft breeze brushes against your skin. As you cross a busy street, a car honks loudly at you, the driver glaring as though you've done something wrong. Your first instinct is to glare back or raise your hands in frustration, but you quickly remind yourself: this is not your burden to carry. You smile gently to yourself and walk on, unbothered.

Soon, you pass a garden where an agitated dog leaps up behind a fence, barking and snarling as you go by. The sound is harsh and jarring, but you step to the side calmly. "It's just doing its job," you think. You imagine the dog's true nature—a loyal companion, perhaps even a playful soul—and choose not to dwell on the aggression.

As you near the cemetery, two children standing by the sidewalk point and giggle as you pass. One of them shouts an immature insult, calling you names. You pause for a moment, considering your reaction. But then you realize: their words are as harmless as the barking dog. Children don't yet understand the weight of their actions. Smiling faintly, you let their comments drift away like fallen leaves caught in the breeze.

Now, at last, you step through the gates of the cemetery. The difference is immediate. The hum of the outside world fades into stillness. The first section is orderly, with well-tended graves adorned with fresh flowers. The air feels reverent, and the quiet invites you to slow your pace.

You walk further, into the older section of the cemetery, where nature has been allowed to reclaim much of the space. The path narrows, becoming less defined as wildflowers spill across the ground in a riot of colors. Poppies, daisies, and bluebells sway gently, their petals catching the light like tiny stained-glass windows. Overhead, ancient trees stretch their branches, their leaves casting intricate patterns of dappled sunlight on the earth below.

This part of the cemetery feels like a secret garden, untouched and timeless. The air here is different—fresher, infused with the scent of wildflowers and damp earth. Birds flit among the branches, and a wood pigeon coos softly in the distance. It's as though time slows, inviting you to pause and simply be.

You make your way to your special spot, a secluded clearing hidden behind a thicket of bushes. How you discovered it, you're not sure, but it feels as though it was waiting for you. A smooth stone, perfectly shaped for sitting, rests in a patch of sunlight. It's small, but it's curve fits your body as though nature herself carved it for meditation.

Settling onto the stone, you cross your legs and rest your hands gently on your knees. The warmth of the sunlight on your skin, the soft rustle of leaves, and the distant hum of bees create a symphony of calm. This is your sanctuary.

Closing your eyes, you take a deep breath, feeling the air fill your lungs and expand your chest. As you exhale, you let go of any lingering tension. Your mind begins to wander back to the encounters of the day—the online comment, the honking driver, the barking dog, the giggling children. Each moment arises in your mind like a ripple on the surface of a still pond.

You picture them now as leaves floating on a slow-moving stream. The sharp words online are a brittle, curling leaf. The honking horn is a bright, jagged leaf, vibrant with emotion. The barking dog is a large, heavy leaf, and the children's insults are small, fluttering ones. Each leaf drifts into view, carried by the current.

You watch them come and go, resisting the urge to reach out or hold on. They are just passing through.

As you sit, a deep realization settles over you: these moments are fleeting. They hold no power unless you give it to them. The stream flows on, steady and calm, just as your inner peace remains unshaken.

You breathe in deeply, imagining the sunlight around you filling your chest with warmth and light. This light grows, spreading through your body, radiating outward like a golden glow. It protects you, reminding you that your peace is yours to keep.

Here, in this hidden sanctuary, surrounded by nature's beauty, you feel a profound sense of gratitude. Gratitude for the strength to rise above, to let go of what doesn't serve you, and to choose compassion; for yourself and others.

Take another deep breath, letting this sense of calm and clarity sink deeply into your heart. Know that you can carry this peace with you, no matter what leaves may drift onto your stream in the future. You are the stream—flowing, steady, and free.

XLIX

Savasana III

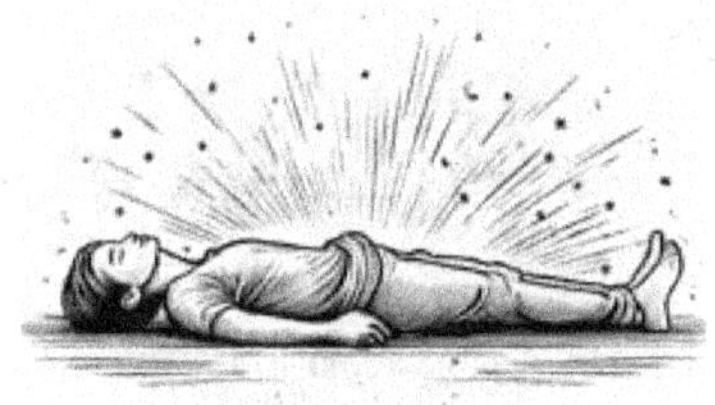

Settle yourself comfortably on the mat, allowing your arms to rest gently at your sides and your legs to relax, open slightly from each other. Feel the mat beneath you, supporting every part of your body. Let yourself sink fully into this place, knowing there is nowhere else you need to be and nothing else to do but simply breathe.

Close your eyes and begin by taking a slow, deep breath in... then gently let it go, feeling any tension start to melt away. Take another deep breath, filling your chest and belly...and exhale slowly, releasing any stress or strain. With each breath, allow yourself to sink deeper into this moment, letting go of the day and inviting a sense of calm to wash over you.

Now, begin to imagine a beautiful, calm ocean stretching out beneath you, warm and inviting. Picture yourself lying back on its gentle surface, floating peacefully on the warm water, feeling completely weightless and free. The ocean cradles you softly, like an embrace, gently supporting every inch of your body as you drift, perfectly at ease. Above you, the sky is vast and clear, an endless expanse of soft blue, meeting the water in a distant horizon.

Bring your attention now to your toes. Feel the warm water touching each one, gently cradling them. Let your toes soften, releasing any tightness, any small stress they may hold. Imagine the water drawing away all tension, leaving only a sensation of warmth and ease.

Allow this feeling to move up to your feet. Feel the arches, the tops, and the heels of your feet relaxing, each part softened by the gentle warmth of the ocean. You can sense the water gently caressing your feet, as though it's soothing away every trace of tightness. Feel your ankles loosen and let go, sinking a little deeper into the warmth.

Now, bring your awareness to your lower legs. Imagine the gentle pressure of the water on your calves, surrounding and supporting them completely. Let each muscle in your calves soften, relaxing deeply, as the warmth moves through them, dissolving any strain. With each exhale, let go a little more, feeling your legs become lighter, as though they're blending with the water.

This calm now flows up to your knees, softening them, releasing any tension in the joints and surrounding muscles. Let the warmth flow around your knees, feeling them relax completely, supported by the gentle cradle of the ocean. Each breath out brings even greater ease, as the water embraces and releases any remaining tightness.

Feel this sense of calm rising to your thighs, allowing each muscle to soften and let go. Picture the warmth spreading through your thighs, soothing every part, from the tops of your legs down to the sides, all the way to the backs of your thighs. With every breath, imagine any tension simply dissolving into the water, leaving you feeling weightless and free.

As you float here, turn your attention to your hips and pelvis. Feel the warmth of the water enveloping this area, soothing any tightness, any strain you may be holding there. Let your hips soften and open, allowing a deep sense of release. Feel any remaining tension gently flowing away, leaving only a sensation of openness and ease.

The calming water now travels up to your lower back, filling this area with gentle warmth and support. Picture each vertebra softening, sinking into the support of the ocean. With each exhale, let your lower back relax even further, releasing any tightness, any effort. Imagine the water taking away any stress, leaving only comfort and peace in its place.

Now, let the warmth move into your abdomen, soothing every part, filling it with a deep sense of calm. Feel your belly soften, any tension melting away as you surrender to the embrace of the ocean. Allow the water to soothe any inner restlessness, creating a sense of calm and stillness. With each breath, you feel lighter, more at ease, as though every cell is filled with peace.

Next, bring your attention to your chest, feeling the warmth rise up to this space. Let each breath fill your chest gently, feeling it expand and soften with ease. The water surrounds you, soothing the area around your heart, allowing it to open and relax. As the water embraces you, let go of any weight or pressure you may be holding, allowing this space to fill with calm and lightness.

Feel this sense of warmth and peace flow into your shoulders now. Imagine the gentle waves of the ocean loosening any tightness there, easing away any burdens or worries. Let your shoulders release completely, dropping down as you surrender to the support of the water. Each muscle relaxes fully, letting go into the warm embrace.

Now, let this wave of calm travel down your arms, easing the muscles in your upper arms, your elbows, and forearms. Picture the warmth flowing all the way down to your wrists, then into your hands. Feel the gentle weight of the water, cradling each hand, each finger, encouraging them to open, to relax completely. Sense the release in every part of your arms, feeling light and free, letting go of anything you no longer need to hold.

Bring your attention now to your neck. Feel the warmth of the ocean rise up, gently supporting your neck and easing any tension there. Allow each muscle to soften, each vertebra to relax as you sink even deeper into the comfort of the water. Feel the back of your head cradled by the gentle waves, completely supported.

Let this sensation of calm now flow up to your face. Feel your jaw softening, your mouth resting easily, as any tension simply melts away. Let your cheeks relax, your eyebrows soften. Feel your forehead smoothing out, every line of stress or worry disappearing into the water. With each breath, let go a little more, feeling your entire face at peace.

Now, allow yourself to be fully embraced by this calm ocean. You are weightless, completely supported by the water, floating in perfect harmony with the earth and sky. The water holds you gently, and you feel a profound sense of connection – to yourself, to the vastness around you. Here, in this moment, you are free from all concerns, from all effort. There is only peace.

Breathe in harmony with the gentle rhythm of the ocean, each breath soft and light, each exhale a release, carrying you deeper into a state of calm. Let yourself drift, knowing you are held, supported, in this endless sea of peace.

When you're ready, gently begin to bring your awareness back, slowly and with ease. Feel the mat beneath you once again, the air around you. Take a deep, grounding breath, letting it fill you with renewed energy. When you're ready, open your eyes, feeling calm, connected, and deeply at peace.

L

Cosmic Connection

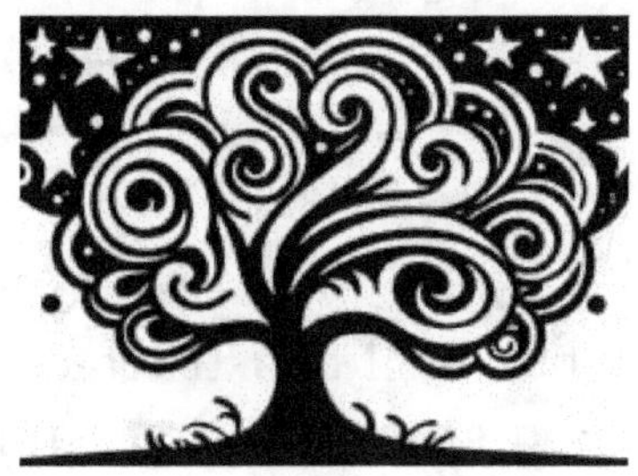

Imagine yourself stepping into a forest at night, surrounded by ancient trees that rise high above, their dark forms casting subtle shadows across the forest floor. The air is cool and crisp, carrying with it the rich, earthy scents of damp soil, pine needles, and fallen leaves. The darkness is thick, enveloping you in a quiet solitude, and you can hear the faint rustling of leaves as a gentle breeze weaves its way through the branches. The forest is alive, yet still; it holds the kind of calm that can only be found under the cover of night, as though the trees themselves are breathing softly, settled into a slow, meditative rhythm.

As your eyes adjust to the low light, you start to pick out shapes and movements in the darkness. An owl calls out in the distance, its low, haunting hoot echoing through the trees, answered by another owl further away, the two in a mysterious dialogue. Bats swoop and dart above you, their tiny wings slicing through the cool night air in silent arcs. Below, you hear the faint rustling of leaves as small creatures—perhaps mice or squirrels—scurry through the underbrush, busy with their nocturnal foraging. It feels like the forest itself is alive, a community of beings thriving in the peace of night.

You're here with a purpose, drawn to this secluded spot to experience something far beyond the ordinary. Slowly, you wander through the trees, guided by an instinct that leads you toward an immense figure in the forest—a tree with a girth and height that set it apart from all the others. Its thick trunk is weathered and ancient, bearing the marks of time and the strength of countless seasons. The roots spread out around it like the fingers of an old giant, weaving deep into the earth, grounding it against the pull of time and elements. You feel a kind of reverence as you stand before it, this guardian of the forest, a living testament to resilience and grace.

On one side of the massive trunk, you notice a sturdy wooden ladder, slightly worn but well-constructed, stretching upwards toward the treetops. You grasp the first rung, feeling the rough wood under your hands, and begin to climb, your movements slow and deliberate. As you ascend, the forest below becomes a shadowy sea, the sounds of nocturnal life gradually receding, replaced by the gentle creak of the ladder and the occasional rustle of leaves brushing against your arms and shoulders.

The ladder winds through thick branches, forcing you to duck and weave as you climb higher, moving in and out of the canopy. Sometimes, the ladder shifts direction as it wraps around the trunk, offering new views of the night-shrouded forest. You pause occasionally to catch your breath, glancing down to see the ground growing farther and farther away, swallowed in shadow. Finally, you reach the top, where the ladder ends at a small platform nestled within the upper branches of the tree, a sort of makeshift treehouse.

The platform is modest, with rough planks and a few canvas panels stretched over one side to form a shelter. It's enough to shield you from the elements if the weather turns, though tonight the sky is clear and inviting, free of clouds. You take a seat on the platform's edge, the night air cool against your skin, and feel an overwhelming sense of calm and anticipation. You've left the forest floor far below, trading the dense closeness of the trees for a breathtaking view of the open sky, a vast expanse dotted with stars.

As you settle in, your eyes turn upward, and the magnificence of the night sky unfolds before you. Stars are scattered like jewels on a dark canvas, each one shimmering with a unique intensity. Constellations you know well come into view, familiar patterns in the endless sprawl of the cosmos. Your eyes are first drawn to Ursa Major, the Great Bear, its form unmistakable as it arches across the sky. Just a short way away, Cassiopeia appears, her elegant "W" shape like a regal signature written across the heavens.

You let your gaze drift toward Orion, the mighty hunter, standing proud in his cosmic pose. Your eyes fall just below the belt of stars, to the faint yet distinct glow of the Orion Nebula, a birthplace of stars nestled in the middle of the universe. You marvel at its faint wisps of light, delicate yet immense, as though a divine hand had painted it in strokes of celestial dust. On a night this clear, you wonder if you can detect a hint of color—maybe the faintest trace of violet or pink. And there, beside Orion, Betelgeuse glows with its deep red hue, an ancient star whose light has traveled through eons to meet your eyes tonight.

Nearby, Venus shines brightly, outshining every other object in the sky. Its light is steady, a beacon against the inky darkness, and you feel a strange sense of companionship with this planet, as though it's watching over you from its place in the heavens. Somewhere nearby, you know that Jupiter and Mars are drifting, and though you don't see them yet, you know you will look for them soon.

For now, though, you simply sit and observe, taking in the splendor of the stars as they quietly shine, just as they have for centuries. You think of those early astronomers, those Arab scholars who studied the stars with only their eyes and gave them names that still echo across the ages. You feel a connection to them, as though you too are part of an ancient tradition, a shared human heritage of wonder and curiosity.

Your gaze shifts to a small, dense cluster of stars high above—

the Pleiades. Known as the Seven Sisters, these stars have been used for generations as a test of eyesight, a measure of clarity and focus. As you try to count each individual star, you feel a thrill of accomplishment, as though you're partaking in a timeless ritual, honoring the brilliance of those tiny, faraway suns.

Eventually, your eyes find Andromeda, the faint smudge of light barely visible against the darkness. It's astonishing to realize that this is not a single star but an entire galaxy, 2.5 million light-years away. The thought fills you with a profound sense of awe. If Andromeda's light were to cease, it would take millions of years for its absence to reach Earth. In the face of such vastness, your own life feels small but strangely significant—a fleeting spark in the great unfolding story of the universe.

The forest around you remains quiet and dark, but then, slowly, you notice a soft glow rising from the horizon. It's the moon, full and orange, casting a warm, diffused light over the landscape. As it rises higher, it shifts to a pale silver, illuminating the treetops and bathing the world in a gentle glow. This is what you've been waiting for, the main event, the celestial body that feels closest to home. The moon's light is so familiar, so deeply comforting. It's easy to forget that it, too, is a distant object, its surface scarred and ancient, forever orbiting Earth in silent companionship.

Lying back on the platform, you gaze up at the vastness above, your body relaxed and your mind quiet, completely absorbed in the beauty of the night. Beneath this star-filled sky, you feel a deep, abiding peace, as though the universe itself is holding you, embracing you in its boundless presence.

As you stare into the night, you're struck by the realization that in this immense cosmos, you are but a small, fleeting existence. Yet, within you, there's a sense of belonging, a sense that you are connected to all of it in ways that are both profound and mysterious. Each atom in your body was born in the heart of a star, and someday, those atoms will return to the universe, continuing the cycle of creation and transformation. In this moment, you understand that you are stardust, a part of the cosmos just as much as the stars themselves.

You lie there, fully present, feeling a sense of unity with the universe. Though you are one tiny soul in a vast expanse, you are here, alive, conscious, bearing witness to the beauty of it all. And as you breathe in this peaceful night, you feel a profound gratitude for the privilege of existence, for the opportunity to be a part of this incredible cosmic dance.

In the silence, beneath the canopy of stars, you feel a gentle acceptance, a quiet understanding that life, in all its fleeting beauty, is a gift to be cherished. And here, high above the forest floor, embraced by the universe, you feel at peace.

LI

Steps Towards Discovery

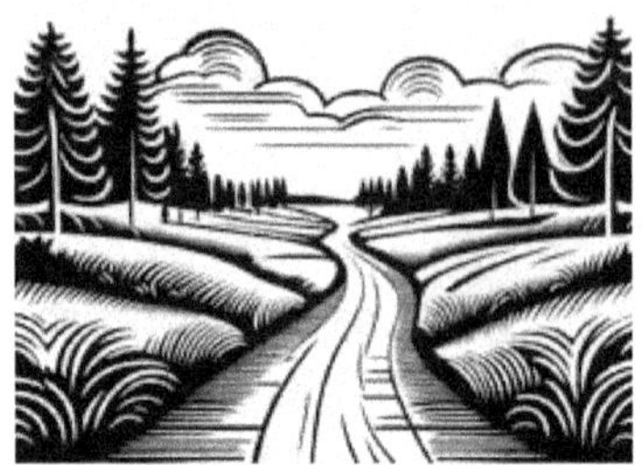

You find yourself standing at the edge of town, right at the dawn of a new journey. All around, there's the familiar chaos of city life—a blur of cars, impatient honks, and the stressed faces of commuters waiting for the lights to change. The faint smell of exhaust lingers in the air. It's rush hour, and you watch as people, each one with their own destination, flow down the street like a fast-moving river. They're caught up in the urgency of daily life, everyone in a hurry to get somewhere.

You pause, feeling a weight lifting from your shoulders as you step onto a quieter footpath. The morning air, brisk and fresh, washes over you. A different energy surrounds you here—one of openness and ease. Almost immediately, you encounter a few people out walking their dogs, who nod in greeting, their faces relaxed and their pace unhurried. It feels like a different world.

The first few hours of walking take you beyond the edges of town, where the narrow streets and buildings fall away. In their place come hedgerows, fields, and the rolling expanse of open countryside. The sights, sounds, and even the air are different here. You catch the faint, sweet scent of wildflowers and listen to the rustle of small creatures hidden in the grass. A hare darts across your path, its movements swift and graceful, disappearing back into the underbrush.

You find yourself slowing down, noticing things that had escaped your attention for far too long. The petals of wild primroses along the path, pale yellow and delicate, seem to glow in the morning light. High above, a kestrel hovers, wings spread wide as it scans the earth below. Every step reveals something new, some small marvel of the natural world that you might have missed in the rush of everyday life.

By evening, you reach a quaint cottage with whitewashed walls, nestled in a small valley. A couple greets you warmly at the door, their faces weathered yet content. They invite you into their cozy home, offering tea and tales of their years spent as potters. Their fingers, roughened by years of shaping clay, tell their own story. You realize that they chose a life of craftsmanship and creativity, a path far removed from the hurried corporate world. It's a reminder of a simpler way of living, one that values time and presence over speed and productivity.

As night falls, you sink into the soft bed they've prepared for you. Your feet are sore from the day's walk, but it's a satisfying ache, a reminder of the journey you're undertaking. Wrapped in the warm quilt, you drift into a deep, restful sleep.

The next morning dawns crisp and clear. After a hearty breakfast, you step back onto the trail. Today's path leads into a dense forest, where towering trees create a canopy overhead, filtering the sunlight into gentle beams that dance across the forest floor. The air is rich with the scent of damp earth and pine, and there's a quiet hush that feels almost sacred. It's like something from an ancient story, a place where each tree holds a thousand secrets.

The forest is alive with sounds—small rustlings as unseen creatures move through the underbrush, the occasional call of a bird echoing through the trees. As you move deeper, the trail narrows, and you catch sight of a few others along the way. Each person you meet exchanges a friendly smile, as if this place draws a certain kind of traveler, one who values quiet conversation and the shared experience of being in nature.

By evening, you find a sheltered spot beneath a sturdy oak to set up camp. Your backpack is light, holding only the essentials. Tonight, you'll sleep under the stars in a simple bivvy bag. As you sit by the small fire you've kindled, the glow flickers over the trees, casting long shadows. The forest has a different feel at night, more mysterious and alive. The hoot of an owl echoes through the darkness, and you catch a glimpse of a fox slipping through the trees, its eyes bright and alert. The crackle of the fire is soothing, grounding you in the present moment. This is solitude, yet you don't feel alone.

The dawn brings a cool mist that drifts through the trees, softening the edges of the world. You wrap yourself in a thick jumper, feeling the chill seep through the fabric. It's a sensation that reminds you of the realness of this journey—unlike the constant, climate-controlled comfort of airports and terminals, this world shifts and changes, and you change along with it.

As you continue, the forest opens up, and soon you find yourself walking along a high cliff overlooking the sea. The waves crash against the rocks below, sending up salty spray. In the distance, the sun rises over the water, bathing everything in a soft, golden light. Gulls wheel overhead, their cries sharp against the backdrop of the ocean's steady roar. The air is filled with the tang of salt, and you feel the vastness of the horizon stretching out before you.

The path leads down to a sandy beach, and you take off your boots, letting your feet sink into the damp sand. The cool, gritty texture is refreshing after days of walking. You spot a small seaside town in the distance and make your way there, savoring the feel of the sand beneath your toes. When you reach the town, you indulge in a plate of fish and chips, watching as people go about their lives at a slower pace than in the city. Here, people smile easily, and there's a friendliness that's a welcome contrast to the hurried anonymity of train stations and airports.

Evening draws near, and you continue your journey along winding roads that lead up into the hills. You find a small inn tucked into the corner of a village, and the innkeeper offers you a room, though she warns it's music night. Grateful for the warmth and the company, you join the gathering downstairs, where locals fill the room with lively conversation. Musicians gather in the corner—a fiddler, a drummer, a penny whistle player, and a guitarist. They play a mix of old folk tunes, their music filling the air with a joyful energy that resonates in your bones.

After a restful night, you set off early, your legs feeling strong and your spirits high. The trail winds upward, and soon you're walking along a rugged ridge, the landscape around you wild and untamed. The hills stretch out in every direction, covered in heather and wild grasses that ripple in the breeze. As you climb higher, the trees thin out, giving way to open moorland, and the wind picks up, sharp and invigorating.

At the summit, you pause to take in the view. The world spreads out below you, vast and open. You meet other hikers at the top, all sharing a quiet sense of wonder at the beauty around them. There's a shared understanding here, an unspoken bond between those who have taken the time to climb to this point.

As evening falls, you reach a mountain bothy—a small stone hut tucked into the hillside. Inside, two travelers have already settled in, a couple from New Zealand and Germany. You share stories over a simple meal, talking by the light of a single candle. The wind howls outside, but inside, there's warmth and camaraderie. You listen to tales of distant lands, of journeys taken and dreams pursued. It's a moment of connection that reminds you of the shared humanity that unites us all.

The final morning dawns bright and clear, with the sun casting a golden glow over the landscape. You descend through a valley, following a path that winds through woods and fields. Along the way, memories surface—moments of frustration from past journeys: a train delayed for hours, a cramped flight with little room to breathe, the faceless rush of people hurrying through crowded terminals. But here, there is a freedom in the simplicity of each step, in the quiet beauty of the land around you.

As you near your destination, you reflect on the journey, on the people you've met, the landscapes you've crossed, and the memories you've made. Each step, each day, has been a part of this adventure, a reminder that life is not about reaching a single endpoint. It's about the path we take, the moments we savor, and the connections we make along the way.

In the end, you realize that this journey has been a celebration of life itself—of the slow, the small, the beautiful details that make each day unique. You walk forward with a sense of peace, knowing that the destination was never the point. It was always about the journey, the simple act of moving through the world, open and aware of the magic in every step.

LII

The Chakras

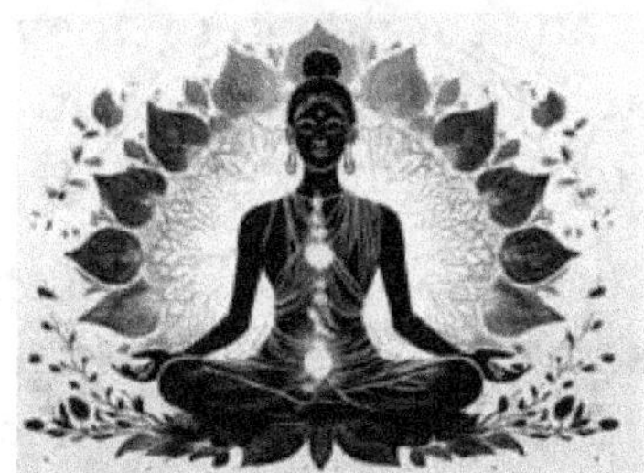

With your eyes closed allow your breath to deepen and your senses awakening to a new realm. You find yourself standing in the heart of an ancient, temperate forest, where time feels as though it has stood still for millennia. Towering trees rise high above you, their trunks thick and gnarled, their bark etched with the wisdom of countless seasons. Moss blankets the base of the trees like a soft green carpet, while ferns unfurl in delicate spirals from the forest floor, their fronds glistening with dew. The air is cool and fresh, infused with the rich, earthy aroma of damp soil and decaying leaves. It smells like life itself.

The canopy overhead is so dense that only fragmented rays of sunlight manage to filter through, casting dappled patterns of gold and green on the ground. This natural ceiling is a mosaic of intertwining branches and leaves, creating a shelter so thick that you can't tell what the weather is like beyond the forest. It feels timeless—untouched by the chaos of the outside world. The undergrowth is alive with sound: the gentle rustle of leaves stirred by an unseen breeze, the distant trill of birdsong, and the occasional creak of wood as if the forest itself were stretching and sighing.

You are completely alone, yet the forest seems to hum with presence, as if the trees, the earth, and the very air are aware of you. This is a place of sanctuary, of quiet connection to something ancient and wise.

A faint path weaves through the undergrowth, barely more than a suggestion of where feet have trodden before. As you walk, the soil beneath you feels soft and forgiving, springy with layers of fallen leaves and pine needles. You follow the path, letting it guide you deeper into the heart of this living cathedral.

Then, you hear it—a sound so subtle at first that you wonder if it's your imagination. A soft hum, deep and resonant, like the faintest whisper of a chant. "LAM." The sound is barely perceptible, but it seems to rise from the very ground itself, growing clearer with each step you take. It feels ancient and powerful, vibrating through the soles of your feet and echoing in your chest. The sound draws you onward, pulling you like a magnet.

As you round a bend in the path, you notice something unusual on the forest floor. Amid the green moss and brown earth lies a stone, dark and gleaming. You kneel to inspect it. The stone is smooth, almost polished, and seems to glow faintly in the dim light. It could be obsidian, with its black glassy sheen, or hematite, with its metallic red undertones. You can't quite tell, but its presence feels significant—important.

You reach out and pick it up. It feels cool and heavy in your hand, its weight grounding and comforting. As you hold it, the stone begins to emit a soft reddish glow, its light pulsing gently like a heartbeat. The glow seems to spread, radiating warmth through your palm and up your arm.

The stone feels alive, as if it's communicating with you, offering you a sense of strength and support. It's as though the stone is saying, *You are safe. You are strong. You belong.* Holding it, you feel a connection to the earth, a deep and unshakable sense of being anchored, much like the roots of the towering trees around you.

Compelled by instinct, you take the stone in one hand and place it against the very base of your spine, where it seems to dissolve into your body. As it disappears, there is a sudden flash of bright red light, vivid and electrifying, illuminating the forest around you for an instant before fading.

In that moment, you feel the energy of the stone settling deep within you. It feels like an anchor, heavy yet reassuring, tethering you to the earth. A profound sense of stability washes over you, as if you are unshakable, rooted like the trees that surround you. You are connected to something timeless and enduring, as if the very ground beneath your feet is lending you its strength.

For a moment, you simply stand there, letting the feeling envelop you. It is a sensation of solidity, of being utterly grounded, and it resonates through every fiber of your being. The hum of "LAM" continues to echo softly, harmonizing with your breath, as the red glow lingers faintly in your awareness—a reminder that you are supported, secure, and deeply connected to the earth.

You take a deep breath, and the forest seems to breathe with you. Inhale, and you feel the cool, fresh air filling your lungs. Exhale, and the trees sway gently, as if nodding in approval. You are ready to continue your journey.

You close your eyes and sense the forest around you fading away, replaced by a warm, golden light. As the light dissipates, you find yourself standing at the edge of a tranquil oasis. The air here feels softer, more humid, and carries the faint, sweet aroma of blooming lotus flowers. Before you stretches a series of shimmering pools, their surfaces reflecting the gentle movements of the breeze like liquid mirrors.

The pools are surrounded by smooth, rounded stones, polished by time and water, glowing faintly under the sunlight. Tiny streams thread through the scene, their delicate trickling sounds creating a soothing harmony that feels almost like laughter in the distance. The water is so clear that you can see the colorful pebbles at the bottom and the darting fish swimming gracefully, leaving ripples in their wake.

A sense of fluidity fills the air—an invitation to let go and flow with the moment. You step closer to one of the pools, the warm earth beneath your feet comforting and grounding. Suddenly, you hear it—a faint but distinct vibration, a melodic hum of VAM, resonating softly. The sound feels alive, playful, inviting, and it seems to be coming from a gleaming object near the water's edge.

As you approach, you see a stone resting on a patch of soft moss. This one glows with a radiant orange hue, smooth and slightly translucent, like carnelian or orange calcite. Its surface feels warm to the touch, its energy pulsating gently, like the rhythm of a flowing stream. Picking it up, you feel an immediate connection —a surge of creativity and emotion. The stone seems to echo with possibilities, inspiring you to dream, to create, to feel.

You instinctively place the stone just below your navel, and it dissolves into your body in a flash of vibrant orange light. A wave of energy ripples through you, as if water were flowing through every part of your being. You feel expansive, open, and free—a river unblocked, moving effortlessly around obstacles.

In this moment, you sense the power of your emotions, not as something to fear but as a source of vitality and inspiration. This is the energy of creation, connection, and pleasure. You breathe deeply, feeling the glow of the stone radiate outward, blending with the warm, creative energy around you.

The sound of VAM grows softer now, blending into the trickling of the streams and the distant rustle of lotus petals. The oasis seems to smile at you, its calm waters reflecting your inner peace. You take one more deep breath, letting this flowing energy settle within you, before turning your attention to the next part of your journey.

The gentle flow of water fades away as the oasis dissolves around you, and you find yourself stepping into a new landscape—a vast, open field bathed in golden sunlight. The air here is warmer, with a dry, invigorating heat that seems to awaken something deep inside you. All around, the tall, golden grasses sway in rhythmic waves, catching the sunlight like strands of spun gold.

Far in the distance, the horizon shimmers as if touched by fire, the golden hues blending seamlessly with bright flashes of orange and yellow. The scent of sun-warmed earth mingles with the faint aroma of wildflowers, creating a heady mix that energizes your senses. Above, the sun burns brightly, not harsh but powerful, its rays descending like golden threads that connect the heavens to the earth.

As you walk through this radiant field, you notice how light your steps feel, as though your body were becoming weightless. You hear it then—a low, resonant hum of RAM, deep and steady, vibrating through the very ground beneath you. It calls to you, guiding your eyes to a small mound of stones in the middle of the field.

You approach and see a stone glowing brilliantly, its surface like polished amber or a fiery citrine crystal. Its color shifts between a bold yellow and golden orange, flickering as if lit from within. The stone pulses with a warmth that grows stronger as you draw closer, radiating an energy that feels both powerful and comforting.

You reach down and pick it up, feeling its heat spread through your palm. It seems to thrum with life, a steady beat that resonates in your chest. Holding it, you are overcome with a sense of confidence, strength, and purpose. It is as though this stone carries the energy of the sun itself, illuminating everything it touches.

Guided by instinct, you press the stone to your solar plexus, just above your navel. As it merges into you, a brilliant golden light bursts outward, filling you with an unstoppable vitality. You feel your inner fire awakening, a strength that has always been there, waiting for you to claim it.

This fire is not chaotic but purposeful; a steady flame that fuels your determination, willpower, and courage. You feel empowered, ready to face challenges and embrace your individuality with pride. This is the center of your personal power, a force that radiates outward, touching everything you do.

The hum of RAM grows softer now, blending into the rustling grasses and the distant whispers of the golden field. You stand taller, your body buzzing with strength and energy, your very being glowing with the light of the sun.

With one final deep breath, you feel the energy settle into your core, a steady flame burning brightly within, as you turn to continue your journey.

The golden field fades away like the warm embrace of a setting sun, and you find yourself stepping into a completely new landscape. This place feels softer, more ethereal, and infinitely expansive. You are surrounded by a lush, emerald-green meadow that seems to stretch endlessly in every direction. The grass beneath your feet is tender, almost velvety, and dotted with thousands of wildflowers in every hue imaginable—delicate pinks, radiant whites, and joyful yellows. Each flower seems to tilt its face toward you, as if welcoming you to this sanctuary of peace.

Above you, the sky is a soothing canopy of gentle blues and soft whites. The clouds drift lazily, their shapes ever-changing, like whispers of compassion floating on the breeze. The air here feels lighter, tinged with the faint aroma of blooming jasmine and roses. A gentle wind stirs, carrying with it the sound of a distant melody—YAM—a resonant, harmonious vibration that seems to echo within your chest.

You walk slowly, taking in the beauty around you. Every step feels like an embrace, every breath like a gift. In the center of the meadow, you notice an ancient tree, its trunk wide and weathered, its branches reaching toward the heavens. Its leaves shimmer in shades of green and gold, and at its roots lies a single stone, glowing softly.

You approach the tree, feeling its quiet strength. The stone beneath it is a soft, translucent green, like jade or aventurine, cool to the touch yet emanating a gentle warmth. Picking it up, you notice how light it feels in your hand, as if it holds the very essence of balance and serenity.

As you cradle the stone, you feel a wave of emotions rise within you. They are not overwhelming, but harmonious; love, compassion, forgiveness, and acceptance. It's as if this stone holds the power to soften the edges of any pain you've ever carried, replacing it with a profound sense of connection to yourself and others.

Guided by intuition, you press the stone to the center of your chest. As it merges into you, a radiant green light spreads outward, washing over you like a warm tide. Your heart feels expansive, open, and limitless, as though it could hold the entire world within its embrace.

You begin to notice how deeply interconnected everything feels —the gentle pulse of the earth beneath your feet, the rustling of leaves in the breeze, the quiet song of the wildflowers swaying in harmony. The energy of this place flows through you effortlessly, dissolving any lingering tension or barriers in your heart.

In this moment, you realize the truth of your own capacity for love; not just love for others, but love for yourself. Forgiveness comes easily here, and the weight of past wounds feels as though it has lifted, replaced by a quiet understanding that you are whole, just as you are.

The hum of YAM resonates deeply, vibrating not only in your chest but in every part of your being. It is a gentle reminder that love and connection are always within reach, no matter the circumstances.

As the green light softens, it settles into a steady glow within your heart, a beacon of compassion and balance that will guide you forward. With your chest light and open, you take a final deep breath, ready to continue your journey with a heart full of warmth and love.

The vibrant green meadow begins to fade, its colors dissolving into a serene, misty blue. The air around you feels cool and crisp, as though you've stepped into a new realm entirely. Before you, an expansive lake stretches out to meet the horizon, its surface so still and clear it reflects the sky above like a flawless mirror. The waters are a soft cerulean, shimmering with hints of silver and deep azure, and the gentle ripple of waves seems to whisper secrets only the wind can understand.

The sky above is endless, an infinite stretch of pale blues, accented by feathery white clouds. High above, birds glide effortlessly, their calls echoing in melodious harmony, as if the entire landscape is alive with sound. The air carries a faint, fresh scent of water, mingled with the cool sharpness of mint or eucalyptus, invigorating your senses with each breath.

You take a step toward the lake's edge, feeling the smooth pebbles beneath your feet. As you walk, you notice the air around you vibrates with a subtle hum, a single resonant tone—HAM— gently weaving through the atmosphere. It's as though the entire environment is singing to you, a soft melody that rises and falls with the rhythm of your own breath.

There, at the shore, you notice a luminous blue stone nestled among the pebbles. It glows faintly, like a drop of the sky captured in solid form. As you pick it up, it feels impossibly light, almost as though it could float away if you let go. Its surface is smooth, cool, and polished, and it seems to pulse faintly with its own energy.

As you hold the stone, you are drawn to place it gently at your throat, just where your voice originates. The moment it touches your skin, it dissolves into you, spreading a wave of light blue energy that flows through your neck, shoulders, and chest. A glowing halo of blue light surrounds your throat, radiating outward like ripples in water.

With this energy comes a sense of freedom—freedom to express your truth, to communicate openly and authentically, and to let your voice be heard. The light opens pathways that had once felt blocked, dissolving any hesitation or fear of speaking up.

You feel the resonance of HAM now, vibrating through your throat and chest, as if your very breath is harmonizing with the world around you. It's not just about speaking; it's about connection—finding your voice and using it to bridge gaps, to share your truth while honoring the truths of others.

As the light settles into a steady glow, you notice the clarity in your thoughts. Words seem to flow effortlessly in your mind, as though every idea and feeling you've ever wanted to express is ready to come forth with ease. You realize this energy isn't just about words—it's about listening too, truly hearing the world and the people around you.

The lake reflects your image, but now you see not only your outer self but the energy within you. Your throat feels open, your voice a powerful tool of connection and expression, and you feel at ease knowing you can communicate authentically and compassionately.

The blue light softens, settling into a calm, steady rhythm, a reminder that your voice is a gift, both to yourself and to the world. With this renewed sense of clarity and expression, you take one last look at the serene lake, ready to continue your journey with truth and openness guiding your path.

As the blue glow of Vishuddha fades into the background, the serene lake and sky dissolve into a twilight landscape bathed in indigo hues. You find yourself standing on a vast, open plateau, high above the world, as if perched on the edge of a mountain. The air here is still and profoundly quiet, holding an almost sacred stillness that feels timeless and infinite.

Above you, the sky is a deep indigo, scattered with stars that shimmer like tiny beacons of light. They seem impossibly close, as though you could reach out and touch them. A crescent moon hangs low, casting a faint silvery glow over the land. The horizon stretches infinitely, blurring the boundary between the earth and the cosmos, leaving you with the sense that you are part of something vast and eternal.

The ground beneath you is smooth and cool, almost like polished stone, with faint patterns etched into its surface; intricate spirals, geometric shapes, and endless mandalas that seem to pulse with an inner light. As you walk, your steps feel lighter, as though the ground itself is supporting you, guiding you toward something extraordinary.

In the distance, you notice a small, luminous shape. As you approach, the hum of OM fills the air, reverberating softly but powerfully through the stillness. It seems to resonate not only around you but within you, vibrating through your very being.

At your feet lies an exquisite indigo stone, sparkling faintly in the moonlight. Its surface is smooth, almost glasslike, and as you lift it, it feels weightless yet substantial, as though it holds the secrets of the universe within it. The stone seems to pulse with a rhythm that matches your own heartbeat, creating a sense of perfect harmony.

You bring the stone toward your forehead, placing it gently at the space between your eyebrows—the seat of your inner vision, your third eye. The moment it touches your skin, it melts into you, sending a wave of deep indigo light radiating outward. The light is cool and soothing, yet it carries an immense power, like the quiet strength of a clear night sky.

The light travels through your mind, illuminating hidden corners, clearing away clutter, and creating a vast, open space. You feel your thoughts slow, becoming calm and focused, as though your mind has been transformed into a serene, reflective pool.

With this clarity comes a heightened sense of perception. You feel as though you can see beyond what is immediately in front of you; beyond appearances, beyond time. It's not just physical sight, but an inner vision that allows you to understand deeper truths, to trust your intuition, and to connect with the wisdom that has always been within you.

The hum of OM grows stronger, resonating through your body, aligning your awareness with the energy around you. You sense the interconnectedness of all things, the threads that weave together the fabric of existence. This realization brings a profound sense of peace and trust, as though you are exactly where you need to be, part of a grand, cosmic design.

The indigo light begins to settle, its energy integrating fully into your being. You feel awake, aware, and deeply connected to both yourself and the universe. Your inner vision is clear, and you trust it to guide you, knowing that the answers you seek are already within you, waiting to be discovered.

With a deep sense of trust and clarity, you take a final glance at the indigo-tinged landscape, ready to move forward on your journey, carrying the wisdom of your intuition with you.

The twilight of the Ajna Chakra fades, and the indigo sky begins to brighten, transforming into a dazzling radiance of pure, white light. You find yourself standing in an ethereal realm, unlike anything you have experienced before—a place where the earth and heavens seem to merge into one seamless, infinite expanse.

There is no ground as you know it, yet you are supported, as though standing on a surface made of shimmering, golden-white light. The air itself sparkles with tiny, luminescent particles, each glowing like a star. The light is soft yet all-encompassing, bathing everything in a sense of peace and purity.

Around you, the space is limitless. There are no walls, no boundaries—only an endless expanse of glowing light and warmth. Above, a radiant lotus flower seems to float, its petals made of pure energy. The petals are countless, layered delicately one upon the other, and they shimmer with iridescent hues— white, violet, and gold merging and dancing together in an eternal rhythm.

As you gaze upward, you hear a subtle, harmonious hum, like the soft vibration of the universe itself. The sound is not external but seems to originate from within, resonating through every part of you, connecting you to the space around you.

On the luminous ground before you lies a small, translucent crystal. It appears to hold the entire spectrum of light within its depths, refracting rainbows as it catches the glow of the lotus above. As you reach down to pick it up, it feels weightless in your hand, yet it emanates an immense energy; a vibration so subtle and refined that it feels like the very essence of life.

You lift the crystal toward the top of your head, where you sense a point of energy just above your crown. As you place the crystal there, it begins to dissolve into light, merging seamlessly with your being. In an instant, a radiant column of energy flows through you, connecting you to the infinite expanse above.

The light from the lotus intensifies, pouring down through the top of your head, cascading like a waterfall through your body. The sensation is indescribable—a complete merging with the universe, a dissolution of boundaries. You no longer feel separate or alone; instead, you are one with the light, with the sound, with everything that is.

In this moment, there is no fear, no doubt, no need. You are weightless, timeless, free. A profound peace washes over you, deeper than anything you have ever known. It is a peace that comes from knowing you are part of something vast, eternal, and loving—a source of infinite wisdom and compassion.

The petals of the lotus above begin to open wider, revealing an even greater brilliance within. You feel yourself drawn upward, as though being gently lifted toward this higher state of being. With each moment, the light within you grows brighter, matching the light of the lotus.

There is no division now between you and the universe. The energy of the Sahasrara Chakra has united you with the infinite, and you understand that this connection has always been there, waiting for you to realize it.

For a moment, time seems to stop, and there is only this—the light, the love, the unity. You rest in this sacred space, allowing the energy to flow freely through you, feeling completely at peace, whole, and perfect.

Gradually, the brilliance begins to soften, as the energy integrates fully into your being. The lotus above remains, a reminder of your connection to this infinite source. You carry its light within you now, knowing that it is always accessible, always guiding you.

With this profound sense of unity and transcendence, you prepare to continue your journey, your spirit elevated, your heart open, and your soul aligned with the infinite light of the cosmos.

As you stand at the culmination of your journey, holding the energies of each chakra within you, you realize that these stones were not mere objects; they were reflections of your inner self, each revealing a facet of the intricate, vibrant being you are. Together, they have awakened a harmony that flows from your root to your crown, grounding you in the earth while lifting you to the infinite. The connection is clear: you are a bridge between worlds, embodying strength, creativity, purpose, love, truth, wisdom, and transcendence. With every breath, you carry this balance forward, a radiant testament to the power of alignment and the beauty of your own infinite potential.

EPILOGUE

As you close this book, take a moment to reflect on the journey we've taken together. Each visualization, each pause to breathe, and each step into the world of imagination has been a journey not just outward, but inward.

This book is not an ending—it's a beginning. Every script, every word, was crafted to be a guidepost, gently pointing you toward your own inner peace, creativity, and strength. As you move forward, remember that the power of visualization is always with you, waiting to be revisited whenever life feels overwhelming or uninspiring.

May you carry the calm of the ocean, the strength of the mountain, the grace of the dancer, and the wisdom of your inner teacher into your daily life. These are not just stories but pieces of you, awakened through the simple yet profound act of imagining.

So as you close this final page, pause. Take a deep breath. Feel the stillness within, the quiet promise of your limitless potential. This is your journey, and it continues with every breath, every step, every moment of stillness.

The next journey isn't in this book.....it's in you!